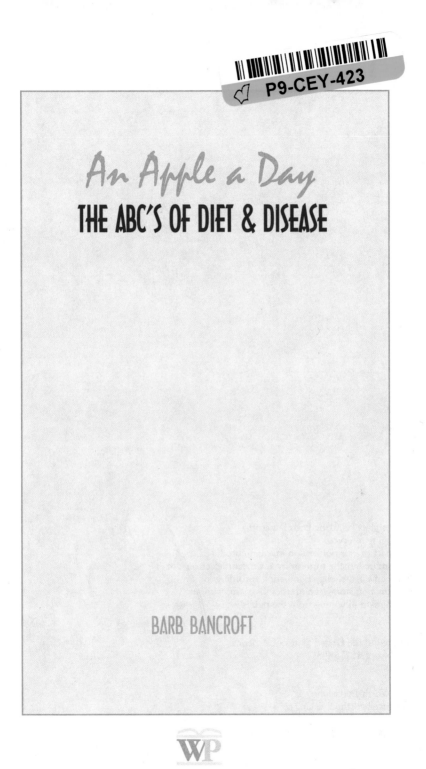

An Apple a Day
THE ABC'S OF DIET & DISEASE

BARB BANCROFT

WP

Printed in the United States of America
ISBN 0-9712776-0-5

WellWorth Publishing
www.wellworthpublishing.com

Book and cover design: Jean Sheldon

Seth

1982-2001

To my beloved Seth kitty,
May your bowl in feline heaven be filled with Fancy Feast.

Thank You

My name as the author may be on the cover of the book, however, an endeavor such as this takes the concerted effort of many friends and colleagues. Thank you all for your suggestions, support and encouragement. To follow the format of the book, I have decided to thank you in alphabetical order.

Ashley. Your drawings are delightful. Best of luck during your next few years in college. I look forward to working with you in the future.

"Bee" Club. Our inspirational Friday night dinners have provided the impetus for many long weekends buried in the books.

Beau, my Dad, and, **Carol,** my Mom. Thank you for always listening to my hair-brained ideas, some of which have worked, some of which have not. Not once have you *ever* discouraged me from trying. (Don't worry, I'm not out of ideas yet!)

Carrie. Thanks for the use of your 24-year old proofreading eyes.

Edy. Whoever you are, I thank you for your low-fat chocolate mint ice cream for sustenance during the long hours slaving over the computer screen.

Gianni. Thank you for taking me on our morning and afternoon walks. They have inspired many a great idea. Your cookie jar will remain full forever.

Ina. How about those delicious recipes? And, that fabulous Chicago restaurant on Randolph Street? Thank you.

Jack. My furry paperweight.

Jake. Thanks for "sleuthing" on the Internet. How do you find everything that I ask you to find? You're the best.

Jean. Since I was so long-winded in the text, I don't have enough space to thank you for all you have done with this book. The cover, the text graphics, your valued opinions, your wit and sarcasm were essential in completing this project. I will give you one week off and then we're starting on the next one. Thank you, thank you, and thank you again.

Jeannine. My appreciation for wonderful food began with you five years ago. Five years later and a few extra pounds in all the wrong places, I still appreciate the fine cuisine that you magically whip up at a moments notice. I look forward to many more years of delicious meals, but hopefully the pounds will not be an accompaniment.

Mary. Did you get a little more than you bargained for this time? What a wonderful editor you have been in the past, present, and hopefuly, the future. (I *still* don't understand that rule about the periods and the parentheses.).

Raemond. Thank you for your continued encouragement. Your opinions and comments are always welcome, solicited or not.

Students and seminar participants. You have all been asking for this for quite some time now. Thanks for continuing to badger, cajole, and encourage me for all of these years.

Contents

Introduction

I think a few explanations are in order before you delve into this compilation of research findings, fun facts, and hysterical/historical highlights.

1) The "average" American. You will notice that I use the term the "average" American often throughout the text. Does such a person exist in the U.S.? No, not exactly. If you have followed the 2000 U.S. Census, you have most likely noticed that the "average" American living in Bemidji, Minnesota is quite different from the "average" American living in Albuquerque, New Mexico. Suffice it to say, the average American is red, yellow, black, and white, male and female, heterosexual, homosexual, asexual, and bisexual, blonde-haired and blue-eyed, black-hair and brown-eyed, blue-haired and cross-eyed. Probably the only commonality we all have as "average" Americans is that we love to eat. When appropriate, I have added gender-based, ethnic-based, and geographically based findings. For the most part, however, we are all the "average" American.

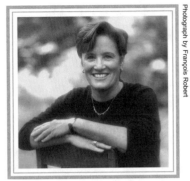

Barb Bancroft
The Average American

Photograph by François Robert

2) The numbers. There are many numbers used throughout this book. These numbers describe amounts consumed, laboratory test ranges, and recommended daily allowances (RDAs) of various vitamins and minerals. I have checked, rechecked, and checked again for the accuracy of these numbers, however, there may be an error hidden somewhere in the text. Please do not hold these numbers as sacrosanct. Always *read the label* of any dietary supplement or multivitamin that you purchase for consumption. Also remember, that just as a teaspoon (tsp.) in a recipe is *not* the same as a tablespoon (Tbsp.), a milligram (mg) is *not* the same as a microgram (mcg).

3) Alphabetical order. All of the headings and subheadings in the chapters are in alphabetical order, with one exception. Each chapter has been given a title, so the text matching the title starts the chapter.

4) Glossary. You will find a glossary (Appendix D) in the back of this book. Words that are green within the body of the text throughout the book, can be found there.

If you have any questions or comments about the book, stop by my web site and drop me a line. Just click on the "Write directly to Barb" button on the home page, and email me. http://barbbancroft.com.

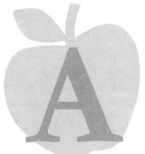

A is for...

An Apple a Day

"An apple a day keeps the doctor away." This proverb comes from the ancient Romans, who believed the apple had magical powers to cure illness. In fact, apples are filled with vitamin C, protein, pectin, natural sugars, copper and iron. The apple's major vitamin contribution to the world of nutrition is vitamin C, the major mineral, potassium. The pectin in the apple is a natural antidiarrheal substance that helps to solidify stool. Shaved raw apple has been used as an herbal remedy for diarrhea and purified pectin has been used as an ingredient in over-the-counter antidiarrheal products. The pectin pushers of the world also claim that it lowers cholesterol by interfering with cholesterol absorption in the bowel.

"An apple a day keeps claustrophobia away." Researchers at the Smell and Taste Treatment Center Foundation in Chicago tested various odors to determine if the odor had any influence on the perception of space. Test subjects found that the smell of green apples made a room appear to be larger than it actually was. The researchers were unable to explain this phenomenon, however, they mentioned that the smell of green apples might be helpful to individuals with claustrophobia.

What is the apple of one's eye? It is the pupil, which in the ninth century was likened to an apple. At that time the eye was believed to be a solid round mass.

Apple juice. Ninety-eight percent of all apple juices sold in the U.S. are pasteurized to stop all natural enzyme action that would otherwise turn sugars into alcohol, eventually producing an alcoholic beverage known as apple cider. Pasteurization also protects apple juice from molds and bacteria such as a deadly strain of colon bacteria found in cows. This bacteria is the deadly *E. Coli O157:H7* (pronounced "Ee co lie Oh, one five seven, aich seven"). Several deaths have been attributed to contaminated unpasteurized apple juices. The unpasteurized apple juice is especially dangerous for children who consume this beverage from roadside stands or homemade apple juice made for yard sales, bake sales and fund-raisers.

The FDA has mandated that a warning be placed on juices that have not been pasteurized. In fact, all juices sold in stores must now be pasteurized.

Can kids get too much fruit juice? The American Academy of Pediatrics (AAP) has updated its 1991 guidelines for juice consumption in kids and recommends the following amounts: *no* fruit juice for infants under 6 months as it offers no nutritional benefit for this age group; limit juice to 4-6 ounces a day for kids 1-6 years old, and 8-12 ounces a day for ages 7-18.

A typical small juice glass holds 4-6 ounces. On average, an 8-ounce serving has 120 calories. Juices that are 100% juice have 11-16 grams of sugar for every 3 ounces, a relatively high amount of sugar. Beverages labeled "fruit drink" are usually almost entirely made of sugar. Consuming large amounts of sugar increases the risk of dental cavities. To protect teeth, the AAP advises parents not to put babies to bed with a bottle of juice. Allowing young children to carry "sippy cups" or boxes of juice around all day also promotes cavities. A second concern is diarrhea and stomach cramps. Much of the sorbitol, the key sugar in juices, is not absorbed in the small intestine, causing abdominal pain and diarrhea if juice is over-consumed. Excess juice is contributing to malnutrition in our children, especially when it takes the place of milk in the daily diet. And last, but not least, the relatively high sugar and caloric load of juice also contributes to childhood obesity.

Appleseed, Johnny. John Chapman (1774-1845), was born in Leominster, Massachusetts and on what should have been his wedding day (his fiance died) in 1797, he left Massachusetts and traveled westward through Ohio, Indiana, Michigan, Iowa and Minnesota to plant apple trees throughout what was then considered "the west." Contrary to popular belief, Johnny did not just "scatter" the seeds as depicted in many stories about his life. Johnny actually was a dedicated nurseryman and helped to establish homesteads for settlers. The law required that each settler plant 50 apple trees during the first year on the homestead. Because of the poor transportation that existed in the "west" in those days, apples were a practical necessity in the early settlers' diets. Johnny Appleseed died on March 18, 1845 in Fort Wayne, Indiana after close to fifty years of travel.

Apple seeds. Apple seeds may be hazardous to your health if swallowed in large quantities. Kids should be especially aware of the apple seed's potential to poison since swallowing only a few seeds can be fatal in small children. Yikes! Why is that? Apple seeds contain amygdalin, a naturally occurring cyanide/sugar compound that degrades into hydrogen cyanide. Don't panic if an adult accidentally swallows an apple seed. One seed is not enough to shut down the mitochondrial oxygen transport system due to cyanide poisoning. However, as mentioned, swallowing only a few seeds can have potentially lethal consequences to a child.

Adam's apple. This eponym refers to the anterior protuberance of the thyroid cartilage, usually seen in men due to the growth of this cartilage at puberty secondary to testosterone. According to *Brewer's Dictionary of Phrase and Fable* the name comes from the superstition that a piece of the forbidden fruit which Adam ate stuck in his throat and caused the swelling. However, there is no mention in the Bible that the so-called forbidden fruit just happened to be an apple. Another interpretation was offered by Professor Alexander Gode in the *Journal of the American Medical Association* (1968; (206):1058). Professor Gode proposed that the Latin term *pomum Adami* ("Adam's apple") is really an early error in translation of the Hebrew *tappuach ha adam*, which means "male bump." The mistake could have easily been made because a single Hebrew word means both "bump" and "apple," and the Hebrew word for "man" eventually became the proper name "Adam."

A
3

Alcohol and Alzheimer's disease. In a report from the World Alzheimer Congress, a Boston study suggests that a regular, moderate intake of alcohol—one to two drinks per day—may have a protective effect against the development of Alzheimer's disease. This conclusion is based on a comparison of people who had the disease with a group of people from the well-known Framingham heart study, matched in age and gender. Compared with these nondrinkers, those who had one or two drinks per day had a 50% lower risk of Alzheimer's disease. Woohoo! Bottoms up! (*Journal of the American Medical Association*, May 2000)

"They tell you that you will lose your mind as you grow older. What they don't tell you is that you won't miss it." —Malcolm Crowley (1898-1989)

Alcohol and cancer. Alcohol intake is associated with an increased risk of a wide variety of cancers—from the oral cavity to the prostate with a few stops in between. Alcohol is on the list of "probable cause" for cancers of the colon, rectum and breast; "convincing cause" of cancers of the mouth and pharynx, larynx, esophagus, liver; and "possible cause" for lung cancer.

Alcohol and hangovers. The liver and stomach metabolize alcohol into acetylaldehyde via an enzyme known as alcohol dehydrogenase (ADH). Acetylaldehyde is metabolized into acetyl coenzyme A and either eliminated from the body or used in the synthesis of cholesterol and fatty acids. The average American can metabolize the alcohol in 13 ounces (400 ml) of wine in approximately five to six hours. If more alcohol is consumed than that amount, the body will have a surplus with insufficient ADH to metabolize the excess. The excess alcohol will accumulate in the blood and interfere with the liver's metabolic functions and the ability of the kidney to reabsorb water. The individual will urinate excessively and lose every electrolyte and mineral known to man, including magnesium, sodium, calcium, and zinc. Lactic acid levels increase and contribute to the feeling of lassitude and malaise. Blood vessels in the dura covering the brain dilate and throb, and the stomach lining is irritated resulting in gastric upset and abdominal pain. The end result is the familiar "hangover." Symptoms will finally dissipate when the body has produced enough additional ADH to metabolize the alcohol "overload" in the bloodstream.

Alcohol and the heart. A report in the September 28, 1994 issue of the *Journal of the American Medical Association* has shed further light on moderate alcohol consumption and a decreased risk in coronary heart disease. Moderate alcohol consumption is known to increase the "good" HDL fraction of total cholesterol, thus offering protection through positive effects on lipid metabolism. This new study also links alcohol consumption with an increase in tissue plasminogen activator (tPA), the thrombolytic enzyme associated with dissolving fibrin clots. This study found that the highest tPA levels were in study participants who consumed two or more alcoholic drinks per day.

How much alcohol is considered to be cardioprotective? Moderate alcohol intake is defined as one 12-ounce beer or one 4-ounce glass of wine or one ounce of hard liquor such as bourbon, vodka, or scotch for women. Men can have twice that amount for cardioprotection. Does that mean that everyone should start imbibing immediately? No, not at all. The health benefits of an alcoholic drink a day are substantially smaller than those offered by exercise and eating right.

Of course, there are many reasons to not drink alcoholic beverages to protect the heart. Two reasons that mind immediately come to are pregnancy and liver disease.

The benefits of alcohol without the alcohol. According to a new study, ten to twelve ounces of pure grape juice per day reduces the stickiness of platelets within 14 days. Grape juice has also been shown to improve arterial vasodilation. Findings are preliminary and must be taken with somewhat of a grain of salt. The makers of Welch's Grape Juice funded the study. The National Institutes of Health, and the American Hospital Association collaborated on the study.

Alcohol and herbs. Many consumers have no idea that alcohol is a common ingredient in many herbal extracts. In fact, some herbal extracts have as much as 55% alcohol. Most herbal preparations sold in health food stores have the alcohol content listed on the label. Read it! This is especially important if you are considering using the herbal product for a child, a diabetic, a patient with liver disease or a recovering alcoholic. Some of the ginseng products sold in convenience, health food and video stores can contain up to 34% alcohol. Of 55 ginseng-containing vials tested by the government, only 7 were alcohol-free. (*Environmental Nutrition*, March 1998)

Alcohol and liver disease. Don't overindulge! Clinically evident alcoholic liver disease is unlikely until the individual has imbibed excessively for at least six to ten years or so. A conservative threshold amount for this level of disease in men is 70-80 grams per day (about 6 ounces of 86-proof liquor, a six-pack of beer, or a 750 ml bottle of wine). A conservative threshold amount for women for this level of disease is 35-40 grams per day.

Alcohol and nosebleeds. Since alcohol is known to have numerous effects on the clotting system, it could be assumed that individuals who imbibe with gusto might have an increase in bleeding problems. A study in the September 10, 1994 *British Medical Journal* confirms this association. Investigators compared 140 patients arriving at the ER with epistaxis (nosebleeds) to 113 age- and sex-matched controls arriving at the ER with other conditions of the ear, nose and throat. All patients were admitted. Alcohol consumption was quantified by questionnaires within a day after admission. Both groups had 34-35% nondrinkers, however the epistaxis group had 45% stating that they were regular drinkers versus the control group with only 30% regular drinkers. Patients in the nosebleed group also had a higher mean alcohol intake of 33 drinks per week versus seven per week for the control group.

Superficial mucous membrane bleeds such as nosebleeds are usually the result of platelet abnormalities. Alcohol has been shown to not only interfere with the ability of platelets to function; it has also been shown to sup-

A
5

press the bone marrow's ability to produce platelets. Patients with significant nosebleeds should be asked about alcohol consumption.

Alcohol: prenatal exposure and adolescent alcoholism. A 14-year follow-up of single-born children examined the role of prenatal alcohol exposure and the subsequent development of alcohol problems in adolescence. In a multivariate analysis, prenatal alcohol exposure was more predictive of adolescent alcohol use than a family history of alcohol problems. The implications of this study are numerous. At the very least it implicates maternal alcohol use as an important risk factor in the development of alcohol use. In addition, prenatal exposure should be examined when studying the potential heredity of alcoholism. And, lastly, this study also adds to the growing literature on the effects of both stress and teratogens (an agent that can disturb the development of an embryo or fetus,) such as prenatal alcohol exposure on behavior that may not be apparent until adolescence or adult life. (Baer JS, et al. "Prenatal alcohol exposure and family history of alcoholism in the etiology of adolescent alcohol problems." *J Stud Alcohol* 1998 Sept; 59:533-43.)

Alcohol and stroke. Since many of the same risk factors associated with heart disease are the same as for ischemic stroke, it stands to reason that a little toddy might actually protect against cholesterol buildup in the major vessels supplying the brain. A little booze goes a long way, as evidenced by the 1999 study published by researchers at New York Presbyterian Hospital-Columbia University that showed that moderate alcohol consumption reduces the risk of stroke due to plaque accumulation in the cerebral arteries. Drinking copious amounts of alcohol (more than seven drinks per day) did *not* protect against stroke. In fact, heavy drinkers, those who consumed more than seven drinks per day, had an increased risk of an intracerebral bleed, also known as a hemorrhagic stroke. The key concept here appears to be *moderate alcohol consumption,* or one to two drinks per day.

Alcohol and teenagers. Parents may not be too astute when estimating how much their teenagers drink. In one Minnesota study, 2.5% of parents said they thought their adolescent children drank about every two weeks, but 29% of the children admitted drinking that often.

"I know a man who gave up smoking, drinking, sex and rich food. He was healthy right up to the time he killed himself." —Johnny Carson

---

Alcohol and ulcers. Researchers in Germany studied 1,785 adults and found that infection with *Helicobacter pylori*—the bacteria that causes stomach and duodenal ulcers as well as stomach cancer—was most common in *non*-drinkers. They also found that as the daily intake of alcohol *increased*, the number of bacteria in the stomach *decreased*. The effect was greatest in wine drinkers, but was prevalent to a lesser degree in beer drinkers. There were too few drinkers of hard liquor in the study to draw any conclusion about the possible antibacterial benefits of Jack Daniels, Jim Beam and other brands of alcohol. However, if you are not a drinker, as you read this blurb, don't start uncorking that wine bottle just to reduce your risk of *Helicobacter pylori*. This would *not* be a clinical indication to imbibe. (*Epidemiology*, July 1999)

Alcohol and women. The former 3:1 male-to-female ratio for alcoholism is narrowing as more women, especially young women, are experiencing more serious problems with alcohol. A survey conducted by the Gallup Organization reports there are 4.5 million women with a drinking problem, 2.5 million who consume at least 60 drinks per month. The alcoholic beverage most frequently consumed by women is wine and the average age at which women start drinking is 13.

Alcoholism is a greater problem physiologically for women than it is for men. Women become intoxicated more easily due to 30% less gastric alcohol dehydrogenase, the enzyme located in the stomach lining that metabolizes alcohol. Since there is less of this enzyme in women, alcohol is absorbed directly through the stomach lining without being metabolized into a more inactive form. This form is more directly toxic to the female heart and liver and women are twice as likely to die of alcoholism-related illnesses (cirrhosis and cardiomyopathy) as are male drinkers of the same age. In fact, the incidence of cirrhosis and cardiomyopathy occurs a full 10 years prior to that of men.

This is a double-edged sword for women. The good news is that moderate drinking, one to two drinks per day, appears to protect against stroke and reduce the risk of heart disease. The bad news is that one to two drinks per day increases the risk of breast cancer due to the metabolism of alcohol into estrogen-like substances by the liver.

A February 1998 study in the *Journal of the American Medical Association* found that among women who averaged one or fewer drinks per day, the breast cancer risk was 9% higher than it was among nondrinkers. This means that one more woman per 10,000 develops breast cancer per year. The current risk is 11 of every 10,000 women; the risk with one or fewer drinks per day would be 12 of every 10,000 women. Among women reporting two to five drinks per day, breast cancer rates rose by 41%. A study of more than 30,000 Italian women, published in the March 4, 1998 *Journal of the National Cancer Institute,* also found a connection between increasing amounts of alcohol and breast cancer. Researchers calculated that slightly more than one drink a day combined with little physical activity accounted for 20% of breast cancer; and more than 40% among premenopausal women.

A new study of 90,000 women demonstrates that for women who drink one to two drinks a day and also take more than 300 mcg (.3 mg) of folate (folic acid) per day, breast cancer risk reverts to that of a nondrinker. Folate is essential for DNA synthesis, and unfortunately, alcohol blocks the absorption of folate. Taking more than 300 mcg overrides the absorption problem, enabling women to maintain its cancer-protective properties. Check your multivitamin and make sure it contains 400 mcg of folate. (*Journal of the American Medical Association*, May 5, 1999)

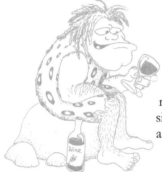

Alcoholism as a by-product of our ancestral nutritional physiology. What's that all about? Sounds like a fancy, convoluted way of making excuses for our overindulgent nature when it comes to imbibing. But, maybe not. Genes for alcohol addiction may have persisted in the human linage for the same reason as those for fat accumulation. Modest amounts of alcohol are known to reduce the risk for heart disease and in turn may lengthen life. Humans predisposed to a little snort may have the survival advantage, and would more likely pass that survival advantage on to their ancestors. This particular genetic trait, most likely useful hundreds of thousands of years ago, is no longer advantageous. Humans no longer have to forage through the underbrush for food and fermenting fruit (sugar/alcohol) to survive. That winning combination can be found in any given corner bar in any given city. (*New England Journal of Medicine*, May 5, 1999)

Are you ready to clean up your act? Head straight to Minnesota, the "Land of 10,000 Treatment Centers," the "Halfway State," or "Minnesober." Located within the state boundaries are 236 outpatient treatment programs, 56 inpatient programs, 46 halfway houses, 35 detoxification centers and 29 extended care facilities. One chemical dependency service estimates that one-half of the 500 patients who enter that facility each year from out of state decide to stay in Minnesober permanently.

Allergies to food. Approximately 33% of Americans believe that they are allergic to certain foods. In reality, 2% of adults and 5% to 8% of children have true food allergies. So, how about all of the folks who think they are allergic to foods? Apparently, every time they eat a certain food they have the classic allergic reaction of itchy or swollen lips, scratchy throat and gastrointestinal upset with cramping and diarrhea.

What's going on then? It appears as if people who are highly sensitive to pollen (a factor outside the food chain), can also experience an allergic response when they eat certain foods that cross react with pollen. Specific foods that can trigger this syndrome, known as oral allergy syndrome (OAS), are celery, tomato, potato, seeds, nuts and fruits. In contrast, the eight foods that trigger 90% of the traditional food allergies are peanuts, tree nuts (e.g. walnuts and pecans), fish, shellfish, eggs, milk, soy and wheat. Cooking food has no effect on the foods that cause traditional food allergies, however, heat usually destroys the protein that cross-reacts with pollen and foods.

Allergies to latex have made a meteoric rise in the past 10 years due to the increased use of wearing latex gloves and using other products containing latex. High-risk groups include healthcare workers, beauticians, and food handlers. Latex, which comes from a certain species of the rubber tree, has proteins that cross react with bananas, avocado, kiwi, water chestnuts, Brazil nuts, and tomatoes. Eating those foods that cross react with latex won't always cause an allergic reaction in latex-sensitive workers, however, it is important to make high-risk groups aware of the problem.

Anaphylactic shock is the top of the line allergic reaction to various foods, drugs, bee stings and even exercise. Anaphylaxis is a life-threatening allergic reaction in which the chest and throat tighten, individuals have difficulty breathing, they turn bright red, and their blood pressure falls to zero. Foods to be aware of include: berries (blackberries, blueberries, raspberries, and strawberries), chocolate, corn, fish, legumes (green peas, lima beans, peanuts, soybeans), milk, peanuts, peaches, pork, shellfish, and wheat.

Food-dependent, exercise-induced anaphylaxis is rare, but may occur after eating a food that usually produces an allergic reaction three to four hours prior to exercising. As they exercise and their body temperature rises, they experience itching, tightness in the chest, and light-headedness. Women are especially vulnerable to this response, so it is advisable not to eat the foods that trigger any reaction within three to four hours of exercising.

A
9

The last potential risk for food allergies exists with genetically modified (GM) foods. The problem for people with allergies is that GM foods may contain allergenic proteins from a different species. Fortunately this is not a huge risk, however, it could be potentially dangerous for super-allergic individuals.

Alpha linolenic acid. Alpha linolenic acid is an omega-3 fatty acid found in soybean and canola oils. Women who eat foods containing high amounts of alpha linolenic acid (particularly oil-based salad dressings and mayonnaise) five to six times per week have a significantly reduced risk of developing fatal ischemic heart disease. Lest one forget—oil-based salad dressings and mayonnaise can be very high in calories, so don't drench the salad in salad dressing because too many calories, even the good omega-3 fatty acid calories, can lead to weight gain. Weight gain in and of itself is a risk factor for heart disease.

Aluminum and Alzheimer's disease. Let's finally put this one to rest, shall we? The first connection between aluminum as a causative factor in Alzheimer's disease was made in the 1970s when Canadian researchers reported that the brains of Alzheimer's patients had over 10 times more aluminum in them than healthy control patients. No studies have duplicated these findings. Cooking with aluminum pots and pans adds only 2.5 mg of aluminum to the daily American diet. By comparison, food additives, like certain leavening or emulsifying agents, add about 10 times that much or 26-50 milligrams. Buffered aspirin contains 125-725 mg, and antacids, 850-5,000 mg. Even with those amounts, no study has proven that aluminum is a cause of Alzheimer's disease. So, that's the aluminum story.

Android obesity. It may come as a surprise to many average Americans, but your waist size should be smaller than your hip size. Android obesity occurs when the waist is larger than the hips and you are shaped like an "apple." Androgens (the male hormone testosterone) tend to move fat around the waist, so men who gain weight tend to pack it right around the paunch.

Once women reach menopause and the ovaries no longer produce estrogen, the adrenal androgens take the opportunity to move fat around the waistline. Can this dreaded complication of menopause be prevented? Yes, by watching what you eat, and by taking estrogen replacement therapy.

A waist/hip ratio can give you an idea if you are creeping toward the apple shape. In a study of over 40,000 middle-aged female nurses, women with a waist-to-hip ratio of greater than 0.88 (apple-shaped) were three times more likely to have a heart attack or die of heart disease over an eight-year period than women with a waist-hip ratio below 0.72 (pear-shaped). (*Journal of the American Medical Association,* December 2, 1998.)

Measure your waist and hips and divide the hip number into the waist number. For women the result should be less than .85 and for men the result should be less than .95.

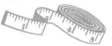

"I'm in shape. Round is shape." —Anonymous

ANOREXIA

Anorexia. Anorexia is the Greek word for loss of appetite. Anorexia is seen in depression, malaise, at the beginning of fevers and numerous illnesses, disorders of the GI tract (especially the stomach) and alcoholism and addiction (especially cocaine). Many medicines have the undesired side effect of causing anorexia and include digoxin and chemotherapy.

Patient had waffles for breakfast and anorexia for lunch.
Note from a patient's hospital chart

Anorexia nervosa. Anorexia nervosa is an eating disorder marked by excessive fasting. It occurs more often in females between the ages of 12 and 21 however it can occur in males and in older females. The individual with anorexia nervosa has an intense fear of becoming obese. This fear does not diminish as weight loss progresses. The patient claims to feel fat even when emaciated. A loss of 25% of the original weight may occur. No known physical illness accounts for the weight loss. There is a refusal to maintain body weight over a minimal normal weight for body and size.

Anorexic pigs. The incessant focus on lean meat and selective breeding has led to a problem that sounds vaguely like an oxymoron—anorexic pigs. A researcher at the University of Wales has identified pigs, typically young females that don't eat enough to maintain their weight. Studies using these pigs may shed some light on possible genetic causes of anorexia and eventually lead to better therapies. (*Nutrition,* July/August 1999.)

Anticoagulants **and food.** Foods that are high in vitamin K may interfere with the effectiveness of anticoagulants such as heparin and warfarin (Coumadin, Dicumarol, Panwarfin). Rich sources of vitamin K include most dark green leafy greens (kale, lettuce, spinach and Swiss chard), asparagus, broccoli, Brussels sprouts, cabbage, cauliflower, and some oils like canola and soybean. Herbal supplements that are known to interact with Coumadin include Dong quai, ginseng, gingko, glucosamine, feverfew, and garlic.

Antioxidants. This is a term thrown around all of the time in clinical nutrition journals, heart journals, cancer journals, and *The Reader's Digest.* Antioxidants are powerful vitamins and chemicals that sop up "oxidants" or "free radicals." In large amounts, the process of oxidation can damage tissues and trigger a chain reaction that deposits cholesterol into the walls of the coronary arteries and cerebral arteries, and that can cause mutations of certain genes predisposing an individual to cancer. So, it only makes sense that "antioxidants" can either prevent these processes or slow them down.

The most potent antioxidants include vitamin C and vitamin E. Extra virgin olive oil contains powerful antioxidants. However, if it loses its "virginity" so to speak, and it is processed to create a milder, "light" olive oil, it also loses its powerful antioxidant property. Carotenoids, the pigments that give many fruits and vegetables their yellow and orange colors, also act as antioxidants. Lycopene a specific carotenoid found in tomatoes, is also a powerful antioxidant that is "unleashed" when the tomato is cooked. Flavonoids are potent antioxidants found in berries—blueberries, raspberries, cranberries, strawberries, and blackberries. Blueberries are number one in this category.

Should you go out and buy those expensive antioxidant formulas that you see on late-night TV? No, that is not necessary. Every nutrition expert in the world concurs that antioxidants are best ingested in produce, if at all possible. The only antioxidant not available in the quantities needed from food sources is vitamin E. Take 200 to 400 IU a day of natural source vitamin E in addition to food sources such as almonds.

Apricots. Ounce for ounce, dried apricots are richer in nutrients and fiber than fresh apricots. It takes five pounds of fresh apricots to make one pound of dried apricots. Drying only removes the water, not the nutrients.

A
12

Dried apricots have twelve times the iron, seven times the fiber, and five times the vitamin A of the fresh fruit. In some studies with laboratory animals, dried apricots have been as effective as liver, kidneys, and eggs in treating iron-deficiency anemia.

The bark, leaves and inner stony pit of the apricot all contain amygdalin, a naturally-occurring compound that degrades to release hydrogen cyanide (prussic acid) in your stomach. Cases of fatal poisoning from apricot pits have been reported, especially in kids mistaking the pits for candy. Extract of apricot pits, known as Laetrile, has been used in the past by alternative practitioners to treat various types of cancer. The presumed mechanism of action is that cyanide destroys the tumor enzyme beta-glucuronidase, an enzyme necessary for cell division. Numerous studies have yet to confirm this mechanism of action and Laetrile has been banned for use in the United States.

Even though Laetrile has not been shown to be effective against established cancers, apricots are rich in beta-carotene and, according to the American Cancer Society they may help to lower the risk of certain cancers of the head and neck, including cancers of the esophagus and larynx.

Artichokes, globe. Vitamin C, iron and potassium are the major contributions to the world of nutrition made by this prickly plant. Some folks are sensitive to the essential oils contained in artichokes and can develop a contact dermatitis from skin contact with those oils. Globe artichokes also contain cynarin, a sweet-tasting chemical that dissolves in water and saliva to sweeten the flavor of anything you eat right after eating the artichoke.

Asparagus. The major contribution to the world of nutrition by the asparagus is its high folate level 131 mcg of folate or 66% of the RDA for a man (current FDA recommendation is 200 mcg) and 73% of the RDA for a woman (current recommendation is 180 mcg for a woman). If a woman is in the mode or the mood to get pregnant the FDA recommends 400 mcg per day to prevent neural tube defects.

Why does eating asparagus make your urine smell funky—kind of like, well, asparagus? The culprit is methyl mercaptan, a compound formed from methionine, a sulfur-containing amino acid found in asparagus. In the past, scientists believed that only people who inherited a certain gene formed the methyl mercaptan, the smelly by-product. Now they think that everyone forms this smelly by-product. However, only a certain number of people inherit the gene that enables them to smell it. (*Environmental Nutrition*, October 1998)

Aspartame (NutraSweet, Equal). Aspartame is a no-calorie sugar substitute found in over 1,500 products. Controversy concerning the safety of aspartame in ongoing, however, most experts agree that it is safe. The one exception is for individuals diagnosed with phenylketonuria (PKU), a rare genetic disease in which the body cannot metabolize the amino acid phenylalanine (a component of aspartame.) A few adverse reactions tend to crop up in small groups of patients and these include headaches, allergic reactions, behavioral changes, and seizures. However, scientific studies have *not* been able to prove a clear connection to the sweetener. And, as to the speculation that aspartame causes brain tumors, there is absolutely *no* scientific basis for an increased risk.

Does this mean that you can drink 27 diet drinks a day containing aspartame? Absolutely not. Even if aspartame is safe, foods that contain the sweetener are usually low in nutrients and should be limited in a healthy diet.

A
14

Aspirin from food. Salicyclates (aspirin) are naturally present in fresh fruit and vegetables. Manufacturers also add salicylates (as antioxidants) to processed foods. Salicylates are also used as antioxidants in cosmetics and are absorbed through the skin. The total amount an average person obtains from these several sources is approximately 125 mg per day, an amount that inhibits platelet aggregation and reduces the risk of myocardial infarction. (By comparison, a "baby" aspirin, or ¼ of a full aspirin, is 82 mg.)

Could this exposure to salicylates via food and cosmetics explain the declining rate of heart disease mortality since the 1960s? Fresh fruit and vegetables did not become available for year-round consumption until the mid-1950s. This was also the same time the manufacturers began adding salicylates to processed foods and long before the average American became diet conscious.

"A rule of thumb in the matter of medical advice is to take everything any doctor says with a grain of aspirin." —Goodman Ace (1899-1982)

Atkins' diet. *Dr. Atkins' New Diet Revolution* claims that carbohydrates (carbs) are the culprits of weight gain. His diet sets strict limits on the amount of carbohydrates one can consume in a 24-hour period. He claims that if you limit carbs, you will burn fat stores. His diet is heavy on meat, poultry, seafood, eggs, cheese, butter, cream, oil, nuts, some (non-starchy) vegetables, and artificial sweeteners. Nutritionally there are some problems with his diet. For starters, the saturated fat content is off the chart. It is also low in fruit, whole grains and fiber, resulting in a major complaint of Atkins' devotees, constipation. Low carbs can also result in a whopping case of halitosis.

One of the reasons weight loss occurs with the Atkins' diet is that less calories are consumed. Interestingly, when one has fewer choices to make, one chooses fewer foods. On average, the high-protein eaters consume about 450 calories less than high-carbohydrate eaters. High protein foods also have a much higher satiety value than high carbohydrate foods. In other words, eating lots of protein is more likely to make you feel full and stop eating.

"I've been on a diet for two weeks and all I've lost is two weeks."
—Totie Fields (1931-1978)

A
15

Avocado. This fruit was introduced to Europe in the early nineteenth century by an Argentinian botanist, Jorge Avocado (1798-1868.) The avocado is an unusual fruit in that 16% of its total body weight is fat, primarily monosaturated fats. The major contribution of the avocado to the world of nutrition is high fiber, vitamins A, folate, and C, and the mineral, potassium.

Because potassium is excreted in the urine, potassium-rich foods are recommended for patients taking potassium-wasting diuretics including furosemide (Lasix), and hydrochlorothiazides (HCTZ). One avocado contains 1,000 mg of potassium. Another benefit of the potassium-rich avocado is the reduction in the risk of stroke. A 1998 Harvard School of Public Health analysis of data from the long-running Health Professionals Study shows 38% fewer strokes among men who ate nine servings of high potassium foods a day versus those who ate less than four servings. Among men with high blood pressure, taking a daily 1,000 mg potassium supplement reduced the incidence of stroke by 60%.

Avocados also contain large amounts of serotonin and may interact with serum tests for a type of endocrine tumor known as a carcinoid that also secretes serotonin. Eating an avocado within three days of this test may give a false-positive reading. Other foods high in serotonin that may also cause a false-positive reading on this test are bananas, eggplant, pineapples, plums, tomatoes, and walnuts.

Apple and Avocado Salad
Serves 6

ina's

breakfast · lunch · dinner

1	apple – cored and diced
1	avocado – peeled, pitted and diced
1/2	cucumber – peeled and sliced thinly
4	cups mixed lettuces
1/4	cup parsley – stemmed and chopped

Combine apple, avocado and cucumber. Add the lettuces and parsley and toss gently.

(Dress with the Lemon-Dijon Vinaigrette in the "V" chapter!)

Nutritional info: 1 serving (undressed!) Calories 79; Total fat 5 gr.; Carbohydrates 7 gr.; Fiber 3 gr.; Sodium 7 mg.

is for...
Beans, Beans, the Musical Fruit

Beans, beans, the musical fruit. Beans are seeds, packed with complex carbohydrates including starch and dietary fiber. They contain indigestible sugars, plus insoluble cellulose and lignin in the seed covering and soluble gums and pectins in the bean. All beans are a great source of the B vitamin folate, and a good source for both the B vitamin pyridoxine (B6) and the mineral iron. The best beans for folate are chickpeas (191 mcg per ½ cup), black beans (129 mcg per ½ cup), pinto beans (147 mcg per ½ cup), navy beans (128 mcg per ½ cup), and the lowly kidney bean (65 mcg per ½ cup). (Source: see Appendix B)

BUYING TIP FOR BEANS: Try to avoid buying dry beans in bulk. The B vitamins, especially B6 are especially sensitive to light and will be destroyed when overexposed to light. If you are going to buy beans from open bins, look carefully for any holes on the bean surface. Bugs love the open bins and will burrow right through the skin and set up house. Beans in bins also may have a few stones thrown in as well as other debris, so pick your beans carefully. Make sure they are smooth-skinned, uniform in size, and evenly colored.

Beans as fiber. The flavonoids are the pigmented compounds in the coating of beans, making up 10% of the weight of the bean. Flavonoids are also the main source of fiber in navy beans, cranberry beans, mottled pintos, great white Northern beans, and black beans. A half-cup serving provides six to eight grams of fiber. The majority of this fiber (75%) is the insoluble type, thought to decrease the risk of colon cancer and other GI problems such as constipation. The other 25% is soluble fiber, which helps to lower cholesterol.

How to "de-gas" the beans. The offending agents in the beans are called oligosaccharides, which are naturally-occurring carbohydrates. Our bodies lack the enzyme necessary to digest the oligosaccharides so the bacteria in our colon perform the task for us. Unfortunately the metabolism by our friendly bacteria results in not so friendly fire, so to speak, and the tell-tale-tail gas is emitted as flatus.

Soaking, draining and rinsing the beans before cooking helps to de-gas the beans. Use the quick-soak method—boil the beans in water for two minutes, then remove from the heat with the cover on and let it sit for two to four hours. After the allotted two to four hours drain and discard the rinse water, rinse again, and cover with fresh cold water (in a three to one ratio of water to beans.) Finally, cook the beans one to four hours depending on the texture of the beans. Acidic foods like tomatoes should be added only after the beans are fully cooked, because acid toughens the beans.

Build up tolerance gradually. The more often you eat beans, the less likely you will suffer gas. For canned beans, drain the liquid off and rinse the beans. By rinsing canned beans several times and pouring off the water, you not only de-gas the beans but you also reduce the sodium content by 40%.

B

18

BACON

BANANAS

Bananas. The banana is the number one selling fruit in the world. The average American consumes 28 pounds of bananas per year. Bananas are shaped like a smile, have no bones, contain no cholesterol, don't leak, have no seeds, come in their own wrappers, ripen off the plant, are fun to play

AN APPLE A DAY

with, come from a giant herb plant, reduce stress, are 99.8% fat free, contain fiber and vitamins, and are a natural diet food.

When the skin of the banana is yellow-green, 40% of its carbohydrates are starch; when the skin is fully yellow and the banana is ripe, only 8% of the carbohydrates are still starch. Ninety-one percent of the starches have been broken down into sugars—glucose, fructose, and sucrose. The high sugar content of the banana makes it a perfect source for a high-energy snack.

A single banana is called a finger, whereas a bunch of bananas is called a hand. "It's the first fruit you eat when you come into this world, and the last fruit you eat on your way out. Bananas appeal to the very young and the very old, especially when a lack of teeth is a concern." Ken Bannister, proprietor of The International Banana Club and Museum. See Appendix B.

The International Banana Association has a helpful hint for the use of banana peels—the inside of a banana peel makes an excellent shoe polish.

B
19

Bananas and latex Allergies. Certain fruits such as bananas, Brazil nuts, chestnuts, kiwi fruit, avocado, and tomato demonstrate cross-reactivity with latex, most likely because of a resemblance to a latex protein component. These foods have been responsible for anaphylactic reactions in latex-sensitive persons, while many other foods, including figs, apples, celery, melons, potatoes, papayas, and pitted fruits such as cherries and peaches have caused progressive symptoms beginning with oral itching.

Bananas and stroke risk. Bananas are packed with potassium. Each banana contains approximately 1,000 mg of potassium. Potassium lowers the risk of having a stroke. *You* make the connection.

"A foodless world would have the disastrous effect of robbing one's initiative. Ambition has no place in a society that refuses its members the opportunity to become top banana." — Fran Leibowitz

Barley. Barley is a grain that is jam-packed with carbohydrates, high in soluble gums and pectins (fiber), and low in fat with not a drop of cholesterol. It is also a good source of folate, the B vitamin that is good for whatever ails you. One of barley's major benefits is to lower the cholesterol via those soluble gums and pectins. How does that happen? A couple of theories on the cholesterol-lowering properties of barley: The first theory is that pectin forms a gel in your stomach that absorbs fats and literally removes them via the GI tract. The second is that the normal bacteria that inhabit the bowel feed on the beta-glucans in the barley to produce short-chain fatty acids, which in turn slow the natural production of cholesterol in your liver. In other words, you stop making your own cholesterol, which is a major contributor to serum cholesterol levels. Barley also contains tocotrienol, another chemical that acts like a mop and slurps up dietary cholesterol.

After barley is harvested, the grain may be left to undergo a natural chemical process known as germination. During this process, the complex carbohydrates change into pure sugar. The grain, now called *malted barley,* is used as the base for several fermented and distilled alcohol beverages—namely beer and whiskey, and, we all know about their benefits.

Basal flatal rate. The basal flatal rate (BFR) is the amount of gas produced as a steady state over a 24-hour period. The average BFR is 15 ml per hour, but would obviously increase exponentially after one consumes a meal. The elimination of gas is proportionate to the amount formed. Under normal circumstances, the average American passes between 200-2,000 ml of gas (flatus) per 24 hours with a mean of 600 ml. This averages out to 13.6 expulsions per day.

Following a basic, standard meal, an increase from 15 ml to 100 ml is observed. This rate is referred to as the post-prandial flatal rate or PPFR. If that meal is comprised of 51% baked beans the PPFR increases to a whopping 176 ml per hour. Now we know why moms only serve baked beans at outdoor picnics.

Beets and beet-red urine. Why do some individuals have beet-red urine after eating beets? It's all in the genes. A pigment in beets, betacyanin, can turn the urine beet-red, but only if you have inherited *both* genes from your parents. The pigment can also cause feces to be bright red, but it will not cause a positive fecal blood test.

Belching. Taking the belch out of soda pop: If you want to lose the carbonation in your soda, pour a room temperature soft drink into a glass of ice. The radical temperature change traumatizes the carbonation ("gas") and you will lose approximately 50% of the carbonation. If you pour refrigerated soda into a chilled glass, you only lose about 10% of the carbonation. Once gas survives the initial impact of meeting the ice in the glass, it doesn't lose carbonation very quickly. Soft drinks with the most carbonation are ginger ale and lemon-lime drinks. Those with the least carbonation are soft drinks with fruit flavors (excluding lemon-lime). Colas and root beer fall in between.

Benecol. Benecol is a margarine substitute that contains plant stanol esters, a chemically altered form of a substance from pine trees. These stanol esters block the absorption of cholesterol in the digestive tract. Benecol also boosts the effects of the "statin" drugs in lowering total cholesterol (by an additional 10-12%) and lowering the LDL cholesterol (by an additional 15-17%). (*American Journal of Cardiology,* July 2000)

B
21

Beverage consumption. The average American consumes a little over 180 gallons of liquids each year: 49 gallons of soft drinks, 33 gallons of water, 23 gallons of beer, and 19 gallons of milk.

Big Mac and super-sized fries. According to a study in *Consumer Reports on Health,* to make up for the calories in just one fast food meal comprised of your basic Big Mac and super-sized fries, you would have to fast for one day and eat nary a drop of fat on the second day.

Speaking of Big Mac Attacks—three new McDonald's "fat" food restaurants come on line every day. McDonald's corporate goal is to have no American more than *four* minutes from one of its restaurants. Seven percent of Americans eat at McDonald's on any given day. McDonald's corporate goal should be to have no American more than *four* minutes away from any coronary care unit.

FACT: One McDonald's Big Mac and large fries = one cup of Crisco, or 1,020 calories and 54 grams of fat. OUCH!

Bilberry (*Vaccinium myrtillus*.) This blackberry is a relative of the blueberry and cranberry. It contains pectins and may be useful for your run-of-the mill basic simple diarrhea attack. Preliminary evidence shows that it may also be helpful in preventing and treating varicose veins, hemorrhoids and eye conditions including diabetic retinopathy, macular degeneration, glaucoma and cataracts. Bilberry also has antioxidant properties that may contribute to its effects, especially those involving ocular conditions. As always, remember that this is preliminary evidence and should be discussed with your health practitioner before indulging.

Clarence Birdseye. Clarence Birdseye worked for the U.S. Government as a surveyor in Labrador in 1912 and 1915. He was investigating the preservation of foods by ice when he wrote, "I saw natives catching fish in fifty below zero weather, which froze stiff as soon as they were taken out of the water. Months later, when they were thawed out, some of those fish were still alive." After his stint with the government, he decided to use the knowledge gained from those frozen fish and start a company that launched individually packaged boxes of peas, spinach, berries, cherries, fish, and meats. In other words, he single-handedly launched the first frozen food products in the United States.

B
22

Blueberries. When it comes to antioxidants, blueberries are your best food source choice. Blueberries placed first over more than three-dozen other fruits and vegetables, including kale, strawberries, spinach and broccoli. What is it about the blueberry that gives it that special antioxidant edge? *Anthocyanin* is the active ingredient that provides such potent antioxidant properties.

Blueberries can also be used as a urinary antiseptic, like cranberries. Blueberries also contain an as yet to be elucidated compound that inhibits the ability of *E. Coli* to attach to the walls of the bladder. If *E. Coli* cannot attach to the bladder wall it cannot trigger a urinary tract infection.

Body Mass Index (BMI). The Body Mass Index is a measure of weight relative to height, making it a crude estimate of body fat. To calculate your own BMI, multiply your weight by 700. Divide that number by your height in inches. Divide that by your height again. What number is staring at your from your calculator? An ideal BMI is 22. A healthy weight is a BMI of 18.5 to 25. An overweight BMI is 25 to 30. An obese BMI is 30 or higher.

What is the average American's BMI? The average American woman is five-foot-four and weighs 152 pounds. That just happens to be a BMI of a little over 25. Her optimal weight is 128 pounds, which would give her a BMI of 22. The average American man is five-feet-nine and weighs 180 pounds. Ideally, he should weigh 150 pounds for a BMI of 22. Oh my. With 97 million Americans overweight or obese, it's tough to get a lean mean population of perfect Americans. And, it's getting tougher all of the time, as the weight of the average American continues to rise.

The risk of chronic diseases starts to rise with certain BMIs. Even though a BMI between 18.5 and 25 is considered to be a "healthy" number, the risk of diabetes starts to rise, especially in women, with a BMI between 22 and 25. Wow. Off we march to Weight Watchers. The risk of heart disease, stroke and most other health problems doesn't climb until the BMI is between 25 and 27. Once you have hit a BMI of 30 or greater, the risk of all diseases skyrockets.

A caveat of importance: BMI is not a useful measurement for children, the frail elderly, serious bodybuilders, or pregnant or breast-feeding women. If your extra weight comes from muscle, not fat, you may have a high BMI even though you're healthy. That doesn't happen to be the case for the average American, however. Also, frail or older people may have a low BMI even though they are unhealthy.

Researchers from the University of North Carolina examined the relationship between age, weight and the risk of dying. They analyzed data from a study that followed more than 300,000 healthy men and women for 12 years. They found that for both men and women between the ages of 30 and 75, those who lived the longest had BMIs between 19 and 22. Having a BMI over 30 almost doubled their risk of dying compared to people of the same age with BMIs lower than 22. (*New England Journal of Medicine*, January 1, 1998).

For more information on how to figure out your BMI see Appendix B.

Botulism. The agent of botulism food poisoning is too small to be seen with the naked eye, yet a 12-ounce glass of the toxin it produces would kill every human being living on the face of the earth, currently 5.9 billion.

Botulism and baked potatoes—a deadly combination. Contrary to popular belief, not all food poisoning due to botulism is due to improper home canning. The CDC (Centers for Disease Control) recently reported on an outbreak of botulism in El Paso caused by infected potatoes that had been baked in aluminum foil.

Potatoes, like all vegetables that are grown underground, can be easily contaminated with *Clostridium botulinum,* the agent that causes botulism poisoning. Washing, scrubbing, and proper cooking can usually kill the spores of *C. botulinum,* however, when potatoes are wrapped in aluminum foil, the foil reflects heat and prevents the potato from getting hot enough to kill all bacterial contaminants. Paradoxically, the heat kills off competing bacteria, making it easier for the *C. botulinum* to grow. Moreover, foil-wrapped potatoes kept at room temperature provide an oxygen-free environment needed for germination of the spores that cause botulism symptoms. (*Environmental Nutrition,* January 1999; *The Journal of Infectious Diseases,* July 1998)

Bread. Bread comes in all shapes, sizes, colors and tastes, from banana nut to pumpernickel to rye to sour dough to whole wheat to just plain old white bread. Even ethnic groups have thrown in their own breads—notably Italian bread, French bread, and Pakistani Tandoori Naan. Each type of bread contains varying amounts of proteins, calories, fats and salt.

Enriched white bread and whole wheat bread are virtually identical as far as the proteins, fats, and carbohydrates contained within, however, white bread has only half the amount of dietary fiber as whole wheat bread. All breads are high carbohydrate foods and are considered to be good sources of B vitamins, including folate. In 1998, the Food and Drug Administration (FDA) mandated that folate be added to flour, rice, and other grain products, which include bread, to help protect against neural tube defects during pregnancy. Bread is a fairly good source of calcium, magnesium, and phosphorus, however, the amounts vary depending on the ingredients used. For example, some bread is made with milk, making the bread a great source of calcium.

All commercially made breads are high in sodium, so if you want low sodium bread you should probably make your own. By making your own bread, you can vary the amounts of salt, sugar, fat and fiber. One missing amino acid from bread is lysine—so it is best to serve foods with bread that

B
24

HISTORICAL HIGHLIGHT

One of the superstitions of the bread world says that if bread does not rise, the devil is hiding in the oven. To protect from the devil, cooks began cutting a cross on top of their loaves to force the devil out and help the bread rise.

In the 1500s bread was served according to status. The working class consumed the burnt bottom of the loaf, the family ate the middle of the loaf, and the guests received the top of the loaf, or the "upper crust."

contain this essential missing amino acid. And, that's easy. Just add milk, cheese, eggs (how about an egg salad sandwich?), meat, fish or poultry.

"Food was a very big factor in Christianity. What would the miracle of the loaves and fishes be without it? And the Last Supper—how effective would that have been?" —Fran Leibowitz

---

One amino acid that is abundant in bread is tryptophan. When you mix the high carbohydrate content of bread with the tryptophan, you get a naturally-occurring calming effect in the brain. The amino acid tryptophan is the major precursor to serotonin in the brain. The carbohydrate helps to "carry" the tryptophan into the brain where it is converted into serotonin, the calming neurotransmitter. This calmness translates to "comfort," so many folks, especially women, will eat lots of bread when they need to be "comforted."

Bread and the Maillard reaction. Impress every one of your friends by telling them that you will be performing a chemical reaction in the kitchen known as the Maillard reaction, named after the French chemist who first identified it. As the drum rolls, the suspense heightens, the group waits with bated breath, two pieces of toast will pop out of the toaster and you will exclaim "Voilá!"

Yes, the Maillard reaction is also known as toasting bread. It is a chemical process by which the sugars and amino acids are caramelized on the surface of the bread, turning it golden brown. One of the side effects of toasting is a change in the nutrient value of bread. The proteins are inactivated and the sugars turn into fiber. However, it remains to be seen as to whether or not the fiber produced by the toasting process has any nutritional value. Some experts are concerned about the carcinogenic potential of toasted bread, however, this should not make you run to the kitchen and toss out the toaster.

"Bread that is sliced with an ax is bread that is too nourishing."
—Fran Leibowitz

BREAKFAST

Breakfast and cognition in school-aged children. Wouldn't it be nice if something as simple as breakfast would save our ailing educational system and flagging student performances? Previous studies have demonstrated that increases in serum glucose improve learning and memory in humans and rodents. The converse is also true in that the lack of nourishment has been shown to adversely affect the cognitive function in school-aged children. A study in the *Archives of Pediatric and Adolescent Medicine* (October 1996), examined the effects of breakfast on short-term cognitive function in children. The study included approximately 500 Israeli children, aged 11-13, from different socioeconomic backgrounds. Two-thirds of the children received a bowl of sugared flakes and a glass of whole milk at school for two weeks, while the remaining children ate their usual breakfast at home or skipped breakfast. Both groups were given a battery of cognitive tests at baseline and after the two-week trial period.

After the two-week trial period, children who ate breakfast at school and tested shortly after scored significantly higher on almost all the tests than children who missed breakfast or who ate breakfast at home one to two hours before the test. There were no differences in test scores between the children who missed breakfast and the children who ate breakfast at home.

It appears as if a burst of glucose shortly before cognitive testing improves intellectual performance. Further studies are needed to evaluate the relative effects of meal content and timing on performance.

"Continental breakfasts are very sparse. My advice is to go right to lunch without pausing." —Miss Piggy

Breakfast of champions. After a good night's sleep, you should "break the fast" with a nutritious and delicious high-powered breakfast to start your day. The best combination to fuel your brain and body is a breakfast consisting of complex carbohydrates (whole grains, fruit), protein (lean meat and dairy), and some fat (margarine, nuts). This combination keeps your blood sugar from skyrocketing and then falling precipitously, and gives you long-lasting energy needed to make it through the hectic morning. Try some of these tasty combinations: Whole grain cereal with skim milk and a big 'ol banana with a smidgeon of peanut butter, or whole wheat pita stuffed with tomato slices and low fat mozzarella cheese zapped in the microwave, or whole grain oatmeal made with low-fat milk and topped with a sprinkling of chopped dates and walnuts. Three taste treats that will get your motor runnin' and keep it hummin' until lunchtime. (Joan Salge Blake, M.S., R.D.)

Breakfast and the blues. Having breakfast on a daily basis helps to keep depression away. Researchers reporting in the *International Journal of Food Sciences and Nutrition* found that adults 20-79 years of age who eat breakfast daily tend to feel less depressed, less stressed, and have lower levels of emotional distress than people who don't eat breakfast every day. In addition, the research showed that persons who eat breakfast also tend not to smoke, drink less alcohol, and follow a healthier diet.

Breast milk fatty acids and IQ tests in infants. Babies fed formula enriched with two fatty acids found in breast milk—DHA (docosahexanoic acid) and arachidonic acid—performed better on tests of mental development than babies fed plain formula. The test used was similar to the IQ test with 100 points being the average score. The mean result for babies fed with the supplemented formula was 105 compared to a score of 98 for the babies fed plain formula. The spread of scores was also an eye-opener: 26% of the infants on the "breast milk formula" scored over 115, compared to only 5% of those on plain formula. Ten percent of the babies on plain formula scored below 85; none in the enriched formula group scored this low. (*Developmental Medicine and Child Neurology,* March 2000)

Broccoli. If you are planning to get your daily calcium intake from devouring broccoli florets, you had better think again. One cup of cooked broccoli (stems and florets) has 70 mg of calcium. Assuming that you are planning on getting all of your calcium from broccoli, you would need to consume approximately 17 cups of broccoli per day.

George Bush, Sr. knows that broccoli is also an excellent source of fiber, vitamin A, folate, and vitamin C, although we have all heard incessantly that it is not one of his favorite foods. It also has a bit of vitamin E and vitamin K. To benefit from all of the vitamins and minerals contained within broccoli, make sure you eat it raw since raw broccoli has up to 40% more vitamin C than broccoli that has been cooked or frozen. Another way to save the goodies in broccoli is to let the water boil for 60 seconds prior to cooking it. Broccoli will lose large amounts of vitamin C if you start cooking it in water that is cold.

Buffet. For the cafeterias and buffet restaurants around the world, we have Pierre Buffet to thank. The seventeenth century Parisian gambler allowed his guests to serve themselves food from a side table. With that the food self-service concept was born and Pierre's name would forever be associated with it.

Bulimia Nervosa ("Hunger like an ox due to a mental disorder.") Bulimia nervosa is an eating disorder characterized by episodic patterns of binge or compulsive eating frequently followed by purging (self-induced vomiting) or other efforts to control body weight such as the use of laxatives and diuretics, and periods of fasting and excessive exercise. Ninety percent of bulimics are females, most often between the ages of 13 and 25. High-risk individuals include teenage girls with a poor self-image who come from a relatively high socioeconomic class. Individuals with bulimia are afraid of becoming fat, however they will consume huge quantities of calories (5,000 to 20,000) during a single binge. Most of the foods consumed are "comfort foods": sweet foods, high in calories, or smooth, soft foods like ice cream, cake, mashed potatoes, pasta, and pastry.

The binge is followed by the purge or by using 20 or more laxatives per day. Patients with bulimia may have problems with dehydration, depletion of essential electrolytes such as hydrogen and chloride from the vomiting or sodium and potassium from the diuretic and laxative abuse. Tooth decay and erosion are common and are caused by regurgitated stomach acid. Excoriation of the back of the first two fingers on the dominant hand is also common due to the self-induced vomiting. Other common findings in bulimics include depression, anxiety, social phobias, or panic disorder. In addition, bulimics tend to engage in other addictive behaviors such as drug or alcohol abuse. Be especially wary of the type 1 diabetic female who presents with wide swings in glycemic control. Some studies have indicated as many as 33-77% are bulimic. These young girls will deliberately withhold their insulin to induce weight loss, resulting in hyperglycemia and diabetic ketoacidosis. Or, they will take their insulin, eat, and then purge. This results in too much insulin for the amount of food absorbed resulting in very low blood sugar, or hypoglycemia. (Rosenthal, M.S. *The Gastrointestinal Sourcebook.* Los Angeles: The Lowell House, 1997)

Broccolini Sauteed with Garlic and Olive Oil

Makes 4 cups

ina's

breakfast · lunch · dinner

4 qts. water	1 Tbsp. Kosher salt
1 lb. broccolini, trimmed	2 tsp. olive oil
3 cloves garlic, minced	

Bring the water to a boil and add the salt and broccolini.

Cook until tender, about 5 minutes, and drain.

Put olive oil and garlic in large pan over medium heat and cook the garlic just until it begins to color.

Add the broccolini and stir for 5 minutes. Serve.

Nutritional info: Serving size 1/2 cup. Calories 54; Total fat 2.6 gr.; Protein 3.5 gr.; Carbohydrates 6.4 gr.; Fiber 3.6 gr.; Sodium 470 mg.

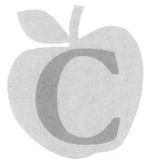

is for...

Chocolate, Chocolate and More Chocolate

Jackie: "Pity there's no such thing as Sugar Replacement Therapy."
Victoria: "There is. It's called chocolate."
—Victoria Wood (1953-:Mens Sana in Thingummy Doodah (1990))

Chocolate is the main by-product of cacao, "The drink of the gods." Cacao is derived from the seeds of a fleshy pod, the fruit of the cacao tree. Chocolate is a plant product and is cholesterol free. Americans are the leading consumers of all forms of chocolate. The Swiss eat the most chocolate per person per day and the Norwegians and Austrians lead the world as the drinkers of chocolate. When consumed in *small* amounts, chocolate can be considered part of a healthy diet, but before you run out and buy a pound of chocolate, be advised that the American Cocoa Research Institute, an arm of the Chocolate Manufacturer's Association, published this morsel of information. The Center for Science in the Public Interest doesn't agree, but here are some chocolate facts so you make the call.

Chocolate does contain saturated fat, however, it is mostly stearic acid, which does not elevate blood cholesterol as much as other saturated fats do. Chocolate does contain other saturated fats, including palmitic acid, which unfortunately, does raise cholesterol. One delicious ounce of chocolate contains 140-150 calories and 9-10 grams of saturated fat. If you add nuts to that ounce of delicious chocolate, add another 20 calories. So, even if chocolate only raises cholesterol slightly, it increases the size of your waist significantly.

Chocolate is rich in antioxidants known as phenolics (like tea and wine) which may protect against coronary heart disease and cancer; one ounce has about as much as a half cup of brewed black tea. Warning—before you make the giant leap connecting a Hershey's candy bar with a reduction in your risk for heart disease, hold off on a few pounds of Godiva until additional data is available. Most likely that will be a long wait, so don't hold your breath thinking that a box of chocolates is cardioprotective. Phenolics in chocolate have not yet been shown to act as antioxidants after absorption. In addition, the "other" ingredients found in chocolate such as saturated fats, sugar, and caffeine may negate any positive effect of the phenolic compounds…oh well, it's worth dreaming about.

Chocolate only has minute amounts of caffeine, and contrary to popular belief, it does *not* cause acne. Chocolate contributes little if any, to tooth decay; plain chocolate bars clear out of the mouth quickly. In addition, cocoa contains tannins, substances that may inhibit dental plaque formation and cavities.

Cocoa powder and chocolate also contain substances that might trigger a cluster of neurons in the limbic system of the brain and produce a feeling of well-being. Cocoa contains several stimulants, including theobromine, caffeine, and serotonin. All three stimulants can provide a little zip to your doo-dah.

Chocolate chip cookies. Ruth Wakefield invented the chocolate chip cookie by mistake in 1930. Mrs. Wakefield was the proprietor of the Toll House Inn, a restaurant located on the toll road between Boston and New Bedford, Massachu- setts. One day, while mixing a batch of chocolate cookies, she ran out of baker's chocolate and substituted pieces of semisweet chocolate in the dough. She thought that the semisweet chocolates would melt in the dough, but much to her dismay, they didn't. And the rest is history—the chocolate chip cookie made its debut at the Toll House Inn—and hence, the original name, Toll House cookies. Chocolate chip cookies remain the most popular cookie in the U.S. where upwards of seven billion are consumed annually. Fifty percent of all cookies baked in American homes are chocolate chip cookies.

Chocolate chip cookies and willpower. How much willpower do you have when it comes to resisting a freshly baked plate of chocolate chip cookies? One study from researchers at Case Western Reserve suggested *not much.* Sixty-seven college students were asked to work alone tracing geometric figures for as long as they could while a plate of freshly baked chocolate chip cookies sat nearby. The students who were allowed to taste the cookies prior to starting the project worked an average of 19 minutes, while the students asked to ignore the cookies gave up after only 8 minutes of toiling away at tracing geometric designs. Apparently the will to resist completely drained the students' self-discipline to continue working.

Chocolate cravings and PMS. Fluctuating hormones in women may trigger chocolate cravings. Peak cravings often appear premenstrually, when estrogen is moderate and progesterone is high. The combination of PMS symptoms and a craving for chocolate may be responsible for a woman's capacity to kill for a bag of M&M's.

CABBAGE

Cabbage and arthritis. Peel off two of the large outer leaves and use a rolling pin to bruise the leaves. Warm the leaves in a microwave, steamer or oven. Wrap the leaves around the painful joints for 15 minutes and repeat the process 2-3 times per day. A similar process can be used for back pain— make a compress with the bruised cabbage leaves and apply it to the painful area of the back for one hour (do not warm the leaves for this application).

Cabbage and breast inflammation (mastitis). Well, if cabbage can do the trick for an "itis" of the joints, it can also do the trick for an "itis" of the breasts...back to the produce department for another head of green cabbage. Nothing like using a head of green cabbage to alleviate the pain and swelling of mastitis in breast-feeding moms. One small randomized trial in the June 1993 issue of *Birth* suggests that the use of cool cabbage leaves reduces the perception of engorgement and more than doubles the likelihood that a patient will still be breast-feeding eight weeks postpartum. Lactation experts recommend using a partially frozen cabbage and peeling the leaves off to wrap around the breast. The leaves are held in place with a brassiere and changed for cooler leaves when necessary.

Cabbage, the Chinese way. Try a few Chinese cabbages if you tire easily of cauliflower and broccoli. There are many varieties of Chinese cabbages and they all have the same health benefits as their cousins in the cruciferous vegetable family. So, to add a bit of variety to your plate, pick up Bok Choy, Chinese Oil Vegetable Cabbage, Napa Cabbage, Shanghai Bok Choy, or Tientsin Cabbage.

CALCIUM

Calcium and...

- **Colon cancer risk reduction.** High fat intake increases fatty acids and bile acids, which are highly irritating to the colon and act as carcinogens. Dietary calcium blocks abnormal cell proliferation and renders bile and fatty acids inert; milk is more effective than supplements. Got skim milk?
- **Decreasing blood pressure—DASH diet.** Two to three servings of low fat or nonfat dairy foods per day is equal to or better than single-drug therapy for hypertension. Food as the source of calcium is two times better than calcium supplements.
- **Decreasing symptoms of PMS.** Women with PMS (premenstrual syndrome, also known as premenstrual dysphoric syndrome) may have an underlying abnormality in calcium metabolism unmasked by fluctuating hormones. Taking 1,200 mg of calcium per day as a supplement has been shown to reduce the symptoms of PMS in some women. Why not give it a try? It certainly couldn't hurt and the extra benefits of calcium for numerous other conditions would be beneficial. P.S. Don't exceed a total of 2,500 mg of calcium per day from food and supplements.
- **Multivitamins.** When purchasing a multivitamin, check out the phosphorus content—the less phosphorus the better. Greater than 100 mg of phosphorus will impair the absorption of calcium.
- **Obesity.** Calcium discourages fat storage and encourages fat breakdown. Got skim milk? (*Federation of the American Society of Experimental Biology,* 2000 June)
- **Osteoporosis.** The typical American diet provides less than 600 mg of calcium per day. The amount of calcium recommended per day to prevent osteoporosis is 1,000 mg if you are between the ages of 19

and 50; 1,200 mg if you are between 51 and 70; and, 1,500 mg if you are greater than 70 years of age. If you don't consume 3-4 servings of low fat milk, yogurt or cheese every day, take a 300 mg calcium supplement for each serving missed.

For more information on calcium and bones:see Appendix B.

Calcium supplements. Calcium and phosphorus compete with each other for excretion by the kidney. Calcium wins if phosphorus is too high. When phosphorus is high, calcium is excreted and the bones can suffer. Foods high in phosophorus also increase calcium excretion. Meat and soft drinks are high in phosphorus. Both increase the risk of osteoporosis. If you want to take calcium supplements instead of eating food that is high in calcium, what type of supplements should you take? Dr. Robert Heaney from Creighton University in Omaha, NE, says what is more important than the type of calcium is to make sure that you get *enough* calcium. In other words, is calcium citrate better than calcium carbonate? Is calcium carbonate better than calcium lactate but not as good as calcium phosphate? Good grief. No wonder the amount consumed is most important. Some rules about calcium consumption:

- Rely on calcium-rich foods first: one cup of frozen yogurt (900 mg); calcium fortified Lactaid nonfat milk (500 mg); one cup of yogurt, non-fat plain (350-400); 1 cup of fat-free or 1% milk (300 mg) for starters.
- If you choose a supplement, take it with meals for maximum absorption. This is especially true with calcium carbonate to avoid gastric distress. Calcium citrate and calcium lactate can be taken between meals.
- Avoid natural sources of calcium like bone meal, dolomite and oyster shell. These may contain toxic amounts of lead, which can lead to cognitive impairment. Read the label for a USP designation. Generally, the products with this designation meet the standards of manufacture, including dissolvability, set by the United States Pharmacopoeia (USP), an independent, not-for-profit group.

C
33

CALORIES

Calories. Just how many calories does the average American need? A person's daily calorie needs depends on many factors, including age, height, weight and activity level. The average goal for most active women, teenage girls and sedentary men is 2,200 per day. If you are a woman and a couch potato, subtract 300-400 calories. As we age we need less calories. Caloric needs decrease 2% per decade for an adult. Older adults and sedentary women need approximately 1,600 calories per day. In other words, at age twenty a cheeseburger and fries doesn't tend to show up on those thighs. At fifty, the cheeseburger and fries make a beeline for those thighs (and hips and waist). If you are an extremely active male or female, you will need more calories. So, here we go. Let's determine each of our caloric needs by following the precise formula found in the July 2001 issue of *Environmental Nutrition*.

Step 1. Determine conversions to kilograms from pounds and centimeters from inches:

Weight in kilograms (kg) = weight in pounds divided by 2.2 (If you weigh 150 pounds, divide that by 2.2 and your weight in kilograms is 68.18 kg)

Height in centimeters (cm) = height in inches multiplied by 2.54 (If you are 60 inches, multiply that times 2.54 and your height in centimeters is 152.4 cm)

Activity factor = 1.2 if sedentary; 1.375 if lightly active 1-3 days per week; 1.55 if moderately active 3-5 days per week; and, 1.725 if vigorously active 6-7 days per week.

Step 2. Determine X, Y and Z:

Women: X = 9.6 times weight in kilograms = _____
Y = 1.8 times height in centimeters = _____
Z = 4.7 times age in years = _____

Men: X = 13.7 times weight in kilograms = _____
Y = 5 times height in centimeters = _____
Z = 6.8 times age in years = _____

Step 3. Determine Basal Metabolic Rate (BMR):

Women: 655 + X + Y + Z = _____
Men: 660 + X + Y + Z = _____

Step 4. Determine Daily Calorie Needs:

Multiply BMR x Activity Factor = _____

To lose one pound per week, subtract 500 from your daily calorie needs; to gain one pound per week, add 500 to your daily calorie needs.

"In two decades I've lost a total of 789 pounds. I should be hanging from a charm bracelet." —Erma Bombeck

---

Caloric intake and the ability to concentrate. The amount that one eats may influence their ability to concentrate. People make more mistakes on tasks that demand sustained attention, such as proofreading, after eating a 1,000-calorie meal compared to a 300 calorie meal, according to research by Angus Craig of the University of Sussex in Brighton, England. Having more or less food than usual also increased errors, although those who ate large meals did much worse as a group. Skipping lunch was not a solution. On an empty stomach, performance fell even lower. People who skipped a meal also felt more tense and anxious. (Lamberg L. *Bodyrhythms.* New York: William Morrow and Company, Inc., 1994.)

Calories still count. Yes, we can all blame a few extra pounds on our parents, or the genetic connection. However, calories still count, unfortunately. Here are the top 10 sources of calories for the consumer in the U.S.: 1) bread, 2) beef, 3) milk, 4) cakes, cookies and doughnuts, 5) soft drinks and soda, 6) poultry, 7) cheese, 8) salad dressing and mayonnaise, 9) margarine, 10) sugars, syrups, and jams.

What is a calorie? Calories are simply a way of measuring the amount of energy supplied to you by the food you eat and drink. The French scientist, Lavoisier, invented the first method of counting calories in the nineteenth century. A calorie is the amount of heat required to raise 4 pounds of water one degree Fahrenheit (or the amount needed to raise 1 quart of water one degree Celcius.) Calorie counting should become a national pastime for the average American. In fact, calorie counting is a necessity for the millions of Americans who must watch their weight. Most dieticians eschew the plethora of fad diets today—the Atkin's diet, The Zone, Sugarbusters, etc. The only way to lose calories, most dieticians advise, is to *cut calories*. Now *that's* a novel concept. In fact, any calories that we don't use to raise that 4 pounds of water 1° F turns to adipose tissue, a fancy way of saying blubber. One measly pound of fat equals 3,500 calories. And yes, you can do the math. That means in order to lose one single pound on the scale you need to burn 3,500 calories. So how can we do that in a painless way?

- Drink 5 fewer beers per week and reduce calorie intake by 700.
- Use two teaspoons of mustard instead of one tablespoon of mayonnaise on your sandwich one time a week and save 90 calories.
- Have one cup of pretzels over the course of one week instead of one cup of nuts and cut 620 calories.
- Use two ounces of fat-free salad dressing instead of two ounces of regular salad dressing (one ounce = two teaspoons) five times per week and save 1,200 calories.
- Use non-stick spray instead of one tablespoon of oil in cooking three times per week and save 330 calories.
- Have a medium piece of fruit instead of two gourmet cookies three times a week and save 1,170 calories.
- A pound is 3,500 calories no matter how you weigh it. Overeat or under-exercise by 200 calories per day and in 17 days you have gained one pound. And the reverse is true. Eat 200 fewer calories per day or burn 200 extra calories per day and you will lose one pound in 17 days.

C
35

Cancer. It is estimated that 10 million people around the world develop cancer every year. Experts estimate that eating healthier foods and getting up off the couch can prevent 30-40% of those cancers. Eating more fruits and vegetables alone could eliminate 20%. (*Nutrition Action,* December 1998.) For a copy of the full 670-page report see Appendix B.

Candy. Just wanted to let you in on a few secrets about candy that we all consume. If you are choosing between a York Peppermint Pattie and Ghirardelli Pure Milk Chocolate, you might want to consider the caloric load of each. The Peppermint Pattie has 170 calories and the Ghirardelli Pure Milk Chocolate has 580 calories. The difference between a 1.7-ounce bag of Peanut M & M's and a 1.7-ounce of Plain M & M's is 10 calories, not enough to spend hours agonizing over the choice. A 4-ounce box of Milk Duds during the movie will set you back 490 calories. Don't substitute the Milk Duds for Junior Mints however. The 5.5-ounce box of Junior Mints is 620 calories.

So, you say, I'll just have the movie popcorn instead. A small popcorn without butter has 400 calories but it's been popped in coconut oil, wiping out a day's worth of saturated fats. An entire large bag of movie popcorn has 1,150 calories, without butter, and 1,650 calories with butter and more than three day's worth of saturated fat. What to choose?

Canker sores. The medically correct term for canker sores is *apthous ulcers.* These benign, albeit painful, ulcers typically occur in the inner surface of the cheeks and lips, but can appear anywhere in the mouth including the tongue, gums, and soft palate. Approximately 20% of the population suffers from occasional canker sores and women are more prone to them than men. The sores usually last between 5 and 14 days.

What causes canker sores? Hypotheses abound, however, the definitive cause remains elusive. Some postulated causes include mouth trauma (hard toothbrushes, dental work, and an accidental chomp to the buccal mucosa), food allergies (citrus and chocolate), nutritional deficiencies (B12, folic acid, iron, and/or zinc), hormonal changes (the ups and downs of estrogen), and immune system impairment. One additional cause discussed in the dental literature is an ingredient found in toothpaste known as SLS, or sodium lauryl sulfate.

From the preceding list it would seem that prevention would focus on eliminating citrus and chocolate from the diet, correcting nutritional deficiencies with multivitamin therapy, and perhaps switching to toothpaste that lacks SLS. After completing that checklist of things to do for prevention, what can you do to treat the existing canker sores? Here are a few helpful hints for soothing the discomfort of the cantankerous canker sore:

- Squeeze a vitamin E capsule onto a cotton swab and apply to the sore for 10 minutes, as needed, to make eating more comfortable.
- Apply licorice in a tincture, powder or tablet of deglycyrrhizinated (DGL) licorice directly to the canker sore.
- Avoid spicy, acidic, and abrasive foods; rinse the mouth with salt water and continue good oral hygiene procedures *even if pain makes it uncomfortable*.
- Over-the-counter topical salves like Anbesol can numb the area temporarily and provide relief for the immediate consumption of a meal.

Canola oil. One of the internet-mediated myths about this heart-healthy oil is that it contains toxins and should not be consumed. This is not true. It contains monosaturated fats and is lower in saturated fats than any other oil except olive oil. So, how did that myth get started?

The myth originates from the fact that canola oil has its origins from a rape plant, a member of the mustard family whose seed oil contains a toxin known as erucic acid. Rapeseed oil is banned in the U.S. because it contains 30-60% erucic acid and can be toxic when used for cooking.

Thirty years ago, Canadian scientists developed a rape plant whose seed oil contained less than 2% erucic acid. This was obviously quite an improvement from the 30-60% found in the older version of the rape plant. They named this plant variety "canola" as a combination of two words—"can" for Canada and "ola" for oil. As of 1990, erucic acid levels in canola ranged from 0.5% to 1%, well under the 2% limit set by our government food police.

Carbohydrate counting. One of the myths that continues to be perpetuated in the world of "sugar" diabetes, is that you can't eat sweets because of the sugar content. This is simply not true, however, before you put this book down and make a beeline for the freezer, please read on.

Carbohydrate counting is more important than reading the label for sugar content. The label still needs to be perused, but look at the serving size and the total grams of carbohydrate. A carbohydrate choice is a serving that equals 15 grams of carbohydrate. For example, *Sunshine Vanilla Wafers* contain *21* grams of carbohydrate in a serving size of 7 cookies. Oops, that's too many carbs for the 15 grams mentioned as a carbohydrate choice. Soooooo, you have to cut back on the number of cookies for *your* serving size. Five cookies would be about 15 grams of carbohydrate, not seven. Put those other 2 *Vanilla Wafers* back in the box for another time.

A nutrition counselor (registered dietician, nutritionist) is an absolute must if you have "sugar" diabetes, or if you are just interested in learning more about healthy eating. This individual can go over choices with you, explain serving sizes, portion sizes, the number of allowable carbohydrate choices, caloric needs for your specific lifestyle, and a myriad of other topics related to health and nutrition. To find a registered dietician see Appendix B.

CARROTS

"Large, naked raw carrots are acceptable as food only to those who live in hutches eagerly waiting for Easter." —Fran Leibowitz

Carrots. One raw carrot, about 7 inches long, has 2 grams of dietary fiber and 20,250 IU of vitamin A (four times the RDA for a man, and five times the RDA for a woman). Carrots are obviously an extraordinary source of vitamin A derived from deep yellow carotenoids (including beta carotene).

Carrots have another claim to fame. Carrots were found to be the most popular food for rectal consumption. Let me explain. The September 1986 issue of *Surgery* published a fascinating review article entitled, "Rectal foreign bodies: Case reports and comprehensive literature review." The literature search found more than 700 identified items that had been removed from no less than 200 rectums, an average of 3.5 items per rectum. Note that those are just the items that could be identified. Who knows how many unidentified flying rectal objects (IFROs) there are out in the "anusphere."

Other foods were also popular. In fact, the rectum was found to be a veritable fruit and vegetable garden. Cucumbers were tied for number one with carrots. Bananas, onions and zucchini tied for the number two spot.

 FACT: Carrots were yellow until a gene mutation created an orange one in the 1700s. An observant farmer appreciated the beauty of the orange carrot and through the process of selective breeding, all of our carrots are now orange.

Celiac disease. Celiac disease is a chronic condition characterized by an inherited sensitivity to gluten (a protein found in wheat, rye, oats and barley). The body's immune response to the gluten produces intestinal damage and in many cases results in chronic diarrhea. In children, celiac disease causes malabsorption of the essential vitamins and nutrients necessary for growth. Children with celiac disease will rapidly improve when all gluten-containing foods are removed from their diet. Gluten should be meticulously avoided for all eternity. Celiac disease in adults presents with all grades of severity, does not always cause diarrhea, and may present in mysterious ways. For example, adults may have recurrent apthous stomatitis (painful ulcers of the gums and tongue), weakness, anemia, osteoporosis, and calcium deposition in the brain with seizures, or the gradual development of dementia. These complications are the result of nutrient deficiencies such as iron, vitamins B12, D, and folic acid, calcium and amino acids. Associated autoimmune symptoms include various "itises" such as dermatitis, arthritis, nephritis, and hepatitis. If you are aware that certain foods always "upset your stomach," causing diarrhea and bloating for days on end, consider testing for celiac disease. Blood tests for gluten antibodies as well as an intestinal biopsy will confirm your suspicions. Once confirmed, call your friendly dietician and read on for hints on changing your diet.

Celiac disease diet. How easy is it to obtain a "gluten-free" diet? It's about as easy as losing 20 pounds for your daughter's wedding by Saturday afternoon. And, it just so happens to be Friday afternoon. When advised to eliminate gluten from the diet, you will be surprised at the number of foods that have the glutens of wheat, rye, oats and barley in them. At least one of the above is present in all prepared foods including most breads, pasta, cookies, cereals, waffles, ice cream, ice milk, candies, chocolate, toffee, meat loaf, sausages, fried chicken, thick soups, sauces, many salad dressings, ketchup, soy sauce, mustard, horseradish sauce, bouillon cubes, curry powder, non-dairy creamer, vinegar, turkey (in its basting ingredients), the filler used in many pills (including over-the-counter drugs), beer, and some types of whiskey. Suffice it to say that *reading labels* is your safest bet for any unknown foods and especially foods that come in boxes, cans, tins, foils, bags, and bottles. Think of the positives—most of the foods you can eat are *fresh*—including fruits, plain meats, eggs, soy, potatoes, corn, rice, broccoli and other fresh vegetables, milk and gluten-free bread (available now at a grocery store in your neighborhood). Consider the advice of a dietician—in fact, call a dietician today. This advice can make all the difference in the world for a symptom-free existence. And, since this diet is part of a treatment regimen, the cost (including mileage) over and above the cost of a normal diet, is tax deductible.

Find several organizations that can offer support in Appendix B.

C
39

Cereal. William Keith Kellogg worked as an assistant to his brother, Dr. John Harvey Kellogg, who was a well-known nutritionist and the director of a hospital specializing in nutritional disorders. In 1884 he discovered a process of making flakes out of grains of maize (corn). These could be eaten as a part of the vegetarian diet recommended by the Seventh Day Adventists, to which sect both brothers belonged. In 1898 the process was industrialized. In 1906 a company was formed to market cornflakes, and ever since then they have been regarded as an integral part of both the English and American breakfast.

"Breakfast cereals that come in the same colors as polyester leisure suits make oversleeping a virtue." —Fran Leibowitz

---

Are all cereals created equal? No, with a capital N. When choosing a cereal, make an attempt to choose one that might be beneficial for your heart *and* your bowels. The key word for both organ systems is fiber, fiber and more fiber. Cereals that contain whole oats reduce the risk of heart disease because of the soluble fiber provided by the whole oats. Cereals that contain *psyllium* can also make the claim that they are "heart healthy" and "bowel movers and shakers." Psyllium is the active ingredient of the over-the-counter laxative, *Metamucil*, used by one and all for bowel cleansing purposes.

Psyllium is the seed husk from the plantago plant. It is a concentrated source of soluble fiber as well as a source of insoluble fiber. When you see soluble fiber, think heart and cholesterol lowering effects; when you see insoluble fiber think bowels and movements. So, psyllium provides that double whammy effect on both ends of the body—top for the heart, bottom for the bowel.

Just a few of the top brands of cold cereal (and this list is not an all-inclusive list, by any means) include:

General Mills *Fiber One Bran* Cereal
Kellogg's *All Bran* Extra Fiber
Kashi *GO LEAN*
Lifestream *Smart Bran*
Health Valley *Organic Apple Crunch* Bran Cereal
Post *The Original Shredded Wheat*
Lifestream *8 Grain Synergy*
Kellogg's Complete *Wheat Bran Flakes*
Erewhon *Fruit 'n Wheat*

Not to be outdone, here are a few top brands for hot cereal:

Arrowhead Mills *4 Grain Plus Flax*
Hodgson Mill *Oat Bran Hot Cereal*
John McCann's *Irish Oatmeal*
Roman Meal *Cream of Rye*
Wheatena
Instant Maypo Oatmeal (maple)

When selecting a cereal, try to find one with at least five grams of fiber and less than eight grams of sugar per serving (16 grams if it contains fruit). Keep an eye on those serving sizes—they can get out of hand when pouring from that big old cereal box. Add some fresh fruit to complete the "color-coded" cuisine. See Color-coded Cuisine later in this chapter.

An important P.S. If you do increase your intake of psyllium, from any source or from multiple sources, you *must* increase your intake of fluids from all sources. If psyllium is taken by itself without extra fluids it has the exact opposite effect on the bowels. Instead of moving those bowels, it stops them in mid-air. Be forewarned.

C

41

CHEESE

Cheese. Did you know that the quality and flavor of cheese is inversely proportional to the thickness of the slice? So when that tightwad neighbor of yours serves you those wafer-thin slices of cheese and you mumble incoherently to no one in particular, "What a cheapskate, skimping on the cheese," he was actually enhancing your taste buds.

To keep the dentist away, eat a chunk of cheese after you finish a meal. At least 12 different types of cheese, including cheddar, mozzarella, Edam, and Gouda, neutralize acids in saliva and help prevent tooth decay. Aged cheddar has also been shown to replenish enamel in decay-weakened tooth surfaces.

The average American consumes approximately 27 pounds of cheese per year. In France, the average person consumes 43.6 pounds of fromage (cheese to the average Frenchman) per year. Over two thousand varieties are produced around the world. If you decided to try a new cheese once a week, it would take just about 40 years to sample all the varieties.

With all of the different cheeses available, does that mean that cheese is a health food? Well, not exactly. Twenty-seven pounds of cheese per year is over a half a pound of cheese per week and cheese is chock full of saturated fat, the bad guy. Each ounce of full-fat cheese contains four to six grams of saturated fat. One yummy slice of a medium size pizza contains one ounce of cheese. Try cutting back to two ounces of cheese per week if you're a "cheesehead." Order your sandwiches, burgers, and salads without cheese and order your pizza with half the cheese. Look for "light" mozzarella, which has half the fat of regular cheese. The mozzarella that says, "part-skim" cuts out only one gram of saturated fat per ounce. Not great, but better than the full-fat cheese.

"If you want to clear your system out, sit on a piece of cheese and swallow a mouse." —Johnny Carson

C

42

Chicken. The average American consumes 50 pounds of chicken per year, as compared to 28 pounds of chicken in 1970.

- **Skin on or skin off?** Should we eat our chicken skinless? When you remove the skin of the chicken prior to consuming you remove two-thirds of the fat. So, if you're trying to cut back on fat and calories, cook it with the skin on, and then remove the skin prior to consumption.
- **Soup, "The Jewish penicillin."** Chicken soup inhibits neutrophils, white blood cells involved in inflammation, hence its anti-inflammatory effects. Of course the hot steam from the soup also helps to break up thick mucus and clear the nasal passages. (Rennard S. *Chest.*, October 17, 2000)
- **White meat versus dark meat?** Leg or a breast? Did the chicken fly across the street or did the chicken walk across the street? The muscles that get the most exercise contain large amounts of myoglobin for oxygen storage. This protein provides a darker color to the muscle, whereas a rarely used muscle will be much lighter in color. Since the majority of our domestic chickens spend little, if any, time in the air, and 99.9% of their time standing or walking, it follows that the leg and thigh are chock full of myoglobin (hence, the dark meat) and the breast and wing are pale in comparison.

Chili peppers. Some of the more common food products made from the various types of chilies are curry powder, cayenne pepper, crushed red pepper, dried whole peppers, chili powder, paprika, pepper sauce, pickled and processed peppers, pimento, and salsa picante. In 1992, the monetary value of sales of salsa picante, a bottled sauce of Mexican origin made with chilies, onions, and tomatoes, overtook that of ketchup in the U.S.

What gives the chili pepper its heat-searing, eye-watering, nose-running, throat-burning wallop? It's called capsaicin (kap-sah-ih-sin), produced by the "placenta" of the pepper, not the seeds. In fact there are a few different kinds of capsaicins and they all have varying degrees of "burn." Three of them cause the "rapid bite," at the back of the palate and throat, and two others cause a long, low-intensity bite on the tongue and the middle palate. Differences in the proportions of these compounds account for the characteristic "burns" of the different types of pepper.

The degree of heat in peppers has actually been measured and documented. This scale is referred to as the Scoville Organoleptic Scale. Your basic mild pepper (the green bell pepper variety) gets a big fat zero on the Scoville Scale. Poblano peppers receive a score of 1,000-1,500; jalapeño peppers have a rating of 2,500-5,000; cayenne pepper rates 30,000 to 50,000; and the hellishly hot Red Savum Habanero scorches in at a walloping 350,000-570,000 Scoville Heat Units. (*Guinness Book of World Records,* 2001)

Clinical uses of chili peppers:
- **Cold feet remedy.** Sprinkle one-eighth of a teaspoon of cayenne pepper into each shoe or glove to generate enough heat to keep the extremities warm. How does it work? The water-soluble components in the cayenne pepper are responsible for vasodilation of the superficial capillaries of the skin surface, resulting in an immediate sensation of heat. Within 15 minutes, oil-soluble compounds reach the deeper layers of the skin, generating warmth for hours. If you're planning to spend at least a few hours out in the frigid cold, perhaps a cayenne liniment is more suitable for keeping the digits warm and cozy. Mix one teaspoon of cayenne pepper with one pint of soy oil in a bottle made of dark glass or opaque plastic. Allow three weeks for the two ingredients to blend, giving the bottle a daily shake. Using a dropper, rub three drops on the soles of the feet, or the palms of the hands. Don't forget to keep your hands away from your eyes after applying the liniment to your hands. Use the liniment only on intact skin. If irritation or cracks occur, run cool water over the affected area and

stop using the cayenne. (Rubman AL, ND, Director of the Southbury Clinic for Traditional Medicines in Southbury, CT.)

- **Fungal infections.** Think *hot* and think *chili peppers* for the treatment of fungal infections. Even though preliminary testing was done on an agar plate, four different concentrations of chopped chili pepper infusions completely wiped out the fungus present in the agar plate. The fungus, *Trichophyton mentagrophytes,* was destroyed even at the lowest concentrations. So keep an eye out for future antifungal agents containing capsaicin.

- **Non-allergic nasal stuffiness.** Researchers at Johns Hopkins Asthma and Allergy Center are experimenting with capsaicin, the chemical that gives hot peppers their zing, as a treatment for chronic, non-allergic nasal stuffiness. Repeated doses appear to clear up nasal passages without permanent damage. One annoying problem—the first few snorts, given ten minutes apart, burned just a tad, and made both the nose and eyes run.

- **Oral ulcers from chemotherapy.** History once again gives us a lesson or two in the treatment of various ailments. In the 1400s, the Aztecs mixed powdered chiles with honey to treat lacerations of the mouth. Oncologists are now capitalizing on this therapy to treat oral ulcers caused by chemotherapy or radiation therapy. Ann Berger of the Yale Cancer Center has mixed a taffylike candy made with capsaicin. When Dr. Berger gave capsaicin-laced candies to 17 patients, 12 of them reported significant pain relief. On a scale from 1 to 10 with 1 being the least pain and 10 being the most pain, ten of the patients rated their pain a 2 as compared to a 6 prior to the candy mixture.

- **Pain of peripheral neuropathy.** Capsaicin depletes peripheral nerves of their supply of substance P, a neuropeptide that sends the message of pain to the brain. Capsaicin is now used to treat pain associated with shingles (Zostrix), rheumatoid arthritis, and "phantom limb" pain.

CHOKING

Choking on foods. What are the five most common foods that cause kids to choke? Hot dogs, candy, peanuts, grapes, and cookies/biscuits.

CHOLESTEROL

Cholesterol. Cholesterol (a lipid or fat) in the blood is coated with proteins called apoproteins. The combination of the lipid with the protein is called a lipoprotein. Lipoproteins come in three varieties—high-density lipoprotein (HDL), low-density lipoprotein (LDL) and very low-density lipoprotein (VLDL). The sum of the three proteins equals the total cholesterol number. HDL is the "good" cholesterol. It picks up the "bad" LDL from the artery walls and transports it to the liver where it is turned into bile and excreted. If HDL-cholesterol levels are too low, LDL continues to pack into artery walls and form fatty plaques.

- The GOOD—HDL levels should be greater than 50 mg/dL (An HDL level of less than 40 mg/dL is considered to be a risk factor for heart disease; optimal levels are greater than 60 mg/dL.)
- The BAD—VLDL levels should be less than 30 mg/dL (This number is calculated by dividing your triglycerides number by 5; if your triglycerides are 150 mg/dL, the VLDL is 30 mg/dL, or 150 divided by 5 = 30...got it?)
- The UGLY—LDL levels should be less than 100 mg/dL (If you have no risk factors for heart disease, or only one risk factor, an LDL of 101 mg/dL to 129 mg/dL is acceptable.)

When considering your risks for heart disease, you need to consider the following: cigarette smoking, blood pressure of 140/90 mmHg or higher, or current use of high blood pressure medication, HDL cholesterol less than 40 mg/dL, family history of premature heart disease in a parent or sibling (before 55 in men, or 65 in women); your age (over 45 in men, over 55 in women), diabetes, and a history of heart disease. (Harvard Heart Letter, August 2001.)

Does everyone need his or her cholesterol lowered? No. It appears as if higher cholesterol levels are beneficial for individuals over the age of 85. The risk of death in this age group decreases by 15% for every 39-point rise in total cholesterol. So, it appears that if you live long enough, cholesterol becomes a friend, not foe.

Autopsies performed on young Americans who died in traffic accidents or by gunshot wounds have revealed that *without exception*, everyone in the 15- to 19-year-old group had roughened areas in their arteries, and 50% had roughened areas in their coronary arteries. The described "roughened" areas are the beginnings of plaque formation and therefore, a fertile soil for the deposition of cholesterol in the arteries. In those who were older than 34 years of age, 50% of the men and 33% of the women had established plaque protruding into the lumen of the coronary arteries.

The implications are quite clear—the pathway to blocked arteries commences early in life. Too many kids are eating their way through every high-fat, high-calorie, fast-food restaurant in America. They are packing their arteries at a ripe young age with pizza, cheeseburgers and "super-sized" fries.

Observing a two-year-old shoving in the fries at McDonalds is an ominous sight to all concerned. Education should start with the parents and continue in the grade school and high school cafeterias where it is all too easy to continue the bad habits that have been established at an early age. (*Journal of the American Medical Association*, 1999; 281:727)

C

45

Cholestin. This over-the-counter dietary supplement is made from rice fermented with red yeast. It's primary claim to fame (and it's a 2,000-year-old claim to fame at that), is its ability to lower moderately elevated cholesterol levels. The active ingredient in red yeast rice is a substance that is chemically identical to one of the "Statin Sisters"—lova, to be exact. Lovastatin is also called Mevacor, a prescription drug for the reduction of cholesterol production in the liver.

Choline and the brain. Rat brains and human brains have similar hippocampuses, the part of the brain responsible for memory. Researchers at Duke University have found that feeding choline to pregnant rats during a critical period of fetal development (the equivalent to the human third trimester when the pathways are being formed in the brain) would significantly improve memory in infant rats. The offspring of rats deprived of choline during this critical period of development showed a marked decrease in their ability to learn and remember information. Since the areas of learning are so similar in the rat and human, researchers are speculating that the same process might occur in humans. Choline appears to enhance pathway formation, essential for neuronal transmission.

The average human consumes less than one gram of choline per day. The average pregnant woman should boost her choline intake in order to provide adequate amounts of the nutrient for the developing fetus. Choline, an amino acid and the building block for acetylcholine, the neurotransmitter of cognition, is found in egg yolks, milk, nuts and liver. Choline is also abundant in breast milk and in some infant formulas. An extra egg or two just might be the difference between a Harvard graduate and the local community college (not that there is anything wrong with that.) Say *Yes* to eggs!! (Swartzwelder S. Duke University Medical Center, Durham, NC)

Chromium. For our bodies to properly use insulin to keep blood sugar levels under control, we need chromium, which we get from food. New research suggests that supplemental vitamins and minerals may help control diabetes or may even help to avert the development of type 2 diabetes. It appears as if some individuals who develop type 2 diabetes are deficient in chromium. Chromium assists insulin in moving glucose into the cells and may help overcome the insulin resistance seen in type 2 diabetes.

The recommended safe and adequate intake of chromium is 50-200 micrograms per day. Most of us in the U.S. get about 50 micrograms from our diet. A study comparing 1,000 mcg of chromium per day with the 200 mcg dose, showed minimal, if any positive benefit from the 200 mcg dose. Chromium is considered a safe mineral and side effects are rare, however, it is not advisable to start taking chromium on your own without discussing it with a health professional. (*Diabetes* 46; 1997.)

Claviceps purpurea is the natural form of LSD (lysergic acid diethylamide), perhaps the most famous hallucinogen of all. It grows, as a fungus on rye, and can cause hallucinations after eating infected rye. Mary Kilbourne Mattosian, a researcher and author on the effects of disease on history, observed that many of the seventeeth century witch hunts (including Salem, Massachusetts) occurred in places where rye was widely cultivated, and after weather that was favorable for the growth of *claviceps purpurea*.

Coca-Cola Classic and the absorption of anti-fungal drugs. The antifungal drugs all have the last name "conazole." For example, itraconazole is Sporanox, ketoconazole is Nizoral, and fluconazole is Diflucan. The "conazoles" absolutely must have an acid environment in the stomach in

C

47

HISTORICAL HIGHLIGHT

In 1886, a pharmacist named John Pemberton was working on his newest concoction in Atlanta, Georgia. He was working on a remedy to relieve exhaustion, aid the nervous tremors, and soothe the headache of a hangover. He mixed his new elixir with a boat oar in a large brass kettle heated over an open fire in his backyard. He took his new elixir to the Jacobs Pharmacy in Atlanta and instructed his assistant to mix the syrup with water and chill it with ice. His assistant accidentally added carbonated water instead of plain water.

They both agreed that the mixture would be a huge success, but not as a hangover remedy. He would advertise it as a fountain drink and an alternative to root beer and ginger ale, the only other two fountain drinks available at that time. He had to come up with a name, so he combined the name of two of the ingredients, coca leaves and cola nuts.

In 1891 another pharmacist, Asa B. Chandler, who had taken Pemberton's elixir for headaches, acquired the rights to Pemberton's formula for a walloping $2,000. Eight years later he set up the franchising system that is the basis of the company's success even today, and put the drink into bottles.

order to be absorbed. The condition known as achlorydia, also known as "the lack of stomach acid," find it impossible to absorb drugs that require this acid environment. Enter Coca Cola Classic—taking an ounce of this brand of soft drink will enhance the absorption of this important class of drugs. Why, you might ask?

The acid content of Coca Cola Classic is similar to that of the gastric acid in the stomach or battery acid in your car for that matter.

FACT: When Coca-cola was first sold as a fountain drink in 1886, sales averaged 9 drinks per day. Today Coca-Cola is consumed in 155 countries with 393 million sold per day.

One 12-ounce can of Coca-cola = 10 teaspoons of sugar (40 grams of sugar.)

Cochineal. Do not skip over this entry just because you have never heard of this word. Cochineal is a red dye made from the pulverized bodies of insects…and you wondered why some drinks, such as Fruitopia, that are colored *red* made *you* red, wheezy, itchy and sneezy. Cochineal has caused severe allergic reactions in individuals with known allergies. After reading this tidbit you may have another type of severe reaction, centered in the organ of nausea, the duodenum. (*Nutrition Action Newsletter,* December 1998.)

Cockroaches and catnip. Researchers from Iowa State University have found that as attractive as catnip is to cats, it's just as repulsive to roaches. Toss a little catnip into a roach-infested cabinet and they scatter as if a nuclear bomb had been dropped in their midst. The only problem is, it doesn't decimate the pesky critters, it only scatters them… but hopefully into the apartment next door.

NOTE: A digression on the dreaded cockroach: "The cockroach's reputation as a filthy creature is undeserved," says Michael Bohdan, professional exterminator and proprietor of The Cockroach Hall of Fame, 2231-B, West Plano, Texas 75075, 972-519-0355. He goes on to state: "They are clean and cautious creatures. They're more careful of where they step with their padded feet than the average person. When I watch them I can see how they react with each other and how they use their antennae to test an area before they walk over it. They groom themselves continually."

Coffee. Coffee was first introduced as a beverage in Arabia around 1,000 A.D. It was called *bunc* and it was believed to be useful as a medicinal tonic. It was finally accepted as a social beverage in the sixteenth century. Napoleon called coffee the "intellectual's drink," Voltaire reportedly drank approximately four gallons of coffee per day, and Bach wrote a sonata, *Coffee Cantata,* as an ode to the drink. Saudi Arabia and Turkey had laws stating that a woman could divorce her husband if he failed to provide her with coffee.

It is estimated that 5,537,000 tons of coffee are produced each year. The average American coffee drinker downs 1.87 cups of coffee per day whereas the average Swedish coffee drinker averages 5.7 cups of coffee per day.

Coffee and blood pressure. It takes four to five cups of coffee to increase blood pressure, not one cup. And the rise in blood pressure is not sustained, therefore it isn't a factor in people who regularly consume caffeine. It's important to realize that the effects of caffeine vary greatly from individual to individual, so blood pressure should be monitored if there is any evidence of an elevation.

C
49

Coffee and caffeine. Each year Americans drink about 127 billion cups of coffee. Twenty-five percent of those cups are decaffeinated.

Speaking of caffeine:
Drip coffee contains 150 mg per 5-ounce cup
Percolated coffee contains 100 mg per 5-ounce cup
Decaffeinated coffee contains 3 mg per 5-ounce cup

Four days after quitting smoking, a person retains 46% more caffeine from a cup of coffee. Why? Cigarette smoking speeds the breakdown of caffeine in the blood, so that smokers need to drink more coffee to maintain their caffeine high.

The *Edinburgh Journal* of 1859 promoted strong coffee as the treatment for asthma. The caffeine in coffee is a potent bronchodilator. Italian researchers found that the caffeine in three cups of coffee had the same bronchodilating effect as a standard dose of theophylline. They also found asthma to be less prevalent among coffee drinkers than non-coffee drinkers.

One day when Winston Churchill was delivering a speech on the floor of the House of Commons, an angry Nancy Astor, the first woman elected to this body stood up and angrily interrupted him. "Winston," she shouted, "if you were my husband, I would flavor your coffee with poison!" Churchill, ever the quick wit with perfect timing replied: "Madam, if I were your husband, I should drink it!"

Coffee and cholesterol. Caffeine is not linked to increased blood cholesterol or LDL-cholesterol oxidation and fat deposition in the arteries. Instead, the culprit called terpenes in coffee is responsible for these unwanted health effects. The good news: using paper or gold filters when you make coffee helps trap the terpenes to keep them out of the cup. However, coffee made with the French plunger or French press, or espresso coffees, including cappuccinos and lattés do contain terpenes.

Coffee and headaches. The headache experienced postoperatively by many patients may have absolutely nothing to do with anesthesia or the surgery—it may simply be due to caffeine withdrawal in patients who have been coffee-deprived 12 hours or more prior to surgery. (Dr. David Danielson, Anesthesiologist, Mayo Clinic 1993)

C
50

Coffee and Parkinson's disease. In retrospective studies, researchers have found that coffee, and possibly tea, are dietary factors whose consumption is significantly less likely in patients with Parkinson's disease as compared with matched controls. In one Japanese study, the risk for developing Parkinson's disease among those who did not drink coffee was double that of those drinking just one to two (4-ounce) cups of coffee per day and was five times greater than the heaviest coffee drinkers (who drank more than seven cups per day).

The molecular basis for this relationship is not known, and of course these findings provide no reason to recommend increased caffeine consumption in order to prevent Parkinson's disease. However, those with a strong family history may consider this as an option. As an extra bonus, the risk for Parkinson's disease is reduced with increased caffeine consumption from any source, including soft drinks and tea. (*Journal of the American Medical Association,* May 2000)

Coffee and suicide in women. A study in the *Archives of Internal Medicine* (1996; 156:521-5) concluded that there was a strong inverse relationship

FACT: One 12-ounce café mocha is the caloric equivalent of one Taco Bell soft taco. It packs a punch with 240-355 calories. Try the café mocha with skim milk and cut the calories by 100.

between coffee consumption and suicide as well as deaths from all external causes of injury, including motor vehicle accidents. The higher the coffee intake, the lower the risk of suicide. (Comment: Depressed individuals may consume coffee to elevate mood, increase energy and their sense of well-being. Non-coffee drinkers may not benefit from this effect.)

"Only Irish offee provides in a single glass all four essential food groups: alcohol, caffeine, sugar, and fat." —Anonymous

---

Coffee enemas for detoxification. Doin' it the old-fashioned way. Nursing textbooks from the 1920s through the 1950s touted the beneficial effects of coffee enemas for a variety of conditions ranging from arthritis to schizophrenia. The *Merck Manual* included coffee enemas as recommended therapy for detoxification until 1977. Coffee enemas were dropped from the *Manual* in 1977 because they had fallen out of fashion with the changing technological advances. Today however, with the re-emergence of complementary and alternative therapies, daily coffee enemas have resumed their place as detoxifying agents in a alternative cancer therapy program known as the Gonzalez/Kelley treatment regimen for pancreatic cancer. In addition, various alternative practitioners favor coffee enemas as a means of enhancing liver function and removing metabolic toxins and waste.

The mechanism of action is presumed to be smooth muscle relaxation of the hepatic ducts resulting in increased secretion of toxins from the liver into the GI tract and out of the body. This only occurs when the caffeine is administered rectally—drinking coffee does not have the same effect on the biliary system.

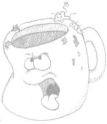

Coffee mugs and disease-causing bugs. Don't assum that your office coffee mug is as clean and tidy as you may think, even though you give it a quick rinse after using it every day. A food safety specialist at the University of Arizona rounded up 53 cups from office kitchens around the campus. Of the 53 cups, 22 were coated with significant numbers of coliform bacteria. Coliform bacteria are those that reside in your colon. This particular group of bugs can wreak havoc in the immunocompromised patient.

And don't forget, looks can be deceiving. Even those coffee mugs that look squeaky clean can harbor a pound or two of the coliform critters. As the investigators continued their search they uncovered the common denominator causing the cup contamination—the dreaded office sponge or dishcloth used to clean all of the cups.

C
51

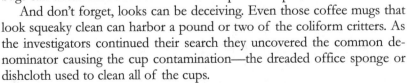

Mugs cleaned with communal sponges or dishcloths were commonly contaminated with the bacteria. Of course, running the sponge or dishcloth through the dishwasher or zapping either of them for a moment or two in the microwave killed all the bacteria. Taking the time to do either one of those bug-bashing activities may present a problem. If time is money, and you have little time, replace the sponge or dishcloth weekly, or clean your mug with a sudsy, disposable paper towel.

Coffee myths. Coffee has been blamed for causing many things, however, very little research substantiates the data. There is no link between heart disease, or pancreatic cancer and coffee. Coffee has no connection with fibrocystic disease. The risk for osteoporosis is questionable, but coffee does not appear to increase the risk, especially when milk is added to the coffee. Coffee has been suspected to increase the risk of miscarriage and birth defects, however, studies haven't supported these claims either. Still, it is recommended that pregnant women drink no more than two cups of coffee per day.

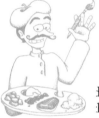

COLOR-CODED CUISINE

Color-coded cuisine. Here's a quick test to see if your diet is diverse enough. Count the colors on your plate. If there are four or more, your diet is "as good as it gets."

COOKBOOKS

"The biggest seller is cookbooks, and the second is diet books…how not to eat what you've just learned to cook." —Andy Rooney

FACT: The Barnes and Nobles web site lists 8,535 cookbooks and 2,782 diet books.

COSMECEUTICALS

Cosmeceuticals. All sorts of dietary products are found in cosmetics today. Read some labels and you'll be surprised to see that cucumber, chamomile, grape seed, pineapple extract, papaya, vitamins C and E, beta carotene, and green tea are just some of the wide variety of nutrients that have been added to cosmetics. Are these nutrients beneficial in the overall scheme of skin care? Evidence for some of the claims made by the companies is just about as scarce as hen's teeth, so don't believe everything you read. Vitamin C may help protect the skin from the sun, but sunscreen does it even better. Vitamin E is rather oily so it may help as a moisturizer, but mineral oil and petrolatum are just as effective at half the cost. Alpha-hydroxy acids (AHA) are derived from milk and fruits such as papaya, pineapple, jojoba, and grapefruit. AHAs have been proven to help with wrinkles and aging spots since they remove the top layer of skin. It's the acid that does the abrasive work and this removal of the top layer of skin can help improve the appearance of the skin. Remember that once the top layer is removed the skin is more vulnerable to the sun, so burning might be an unwanted side effect. And of course, burning results in skin damage, which was probably the reason you were using AHAs in the first place. The vicious cycle continues.

Cows. Did you know that a little less than 50% of the cow is used for beef that is consumed by the average American? However, 99% of the cow is used for various and sundry purposes—in fact, the fine hair from a cow's ear is used as the tip for high-quality paintbrushes for artwork. Beef tallow provides glycerin for cosmetics and toothpaste (vegans beware), soaps, cleaners, shampoos, and detergents. Some of the inedible fats from cattle are used for candles, automobile tires, chalk, crayons, fabric softeners, explosives, ink, and matches. The intestines are perfect casings for sausages and the bones, horns, and hooves have been used for buttons, bone china, glues, animal feeds, piano keys, and fertilizer. It takes the intestines from two cows to provide sufficient "cat" gut to make one tennis racket. Huh? Catgut is a misnomer that took hold over 200 years ago. At that time, sheep intestines were used to make violin strings. As the tale goes, the instrument sounded like a cat screeching, and this became the generic term for natural animal gut. Some of the edible by-products from the cow find their way into some margarines and shortenings and have been used for making chewing gums and candies. Beef by-products have also been used to make drugs, such as beef insulin used by diabetics in the past, glucagon for hypoglycemia, and thrombin to promote blood coagulation during surgical procedures.

FACT: A cow needs three pounds of water to make one gallon of milk.

Cracker Jack. The most important part of a box of Cracker Jack is the toy. The toy was added to each box of Cracker Jack in 1912. Since that time, 17 billion toys have been added to those boxes. In fact, those toys are so important to the image of Cracker Jack, that each packing machine has three electronic eyes aimed at each box to make sure there is a toy contained within. Collectors of all things "Cracker Jack" have valued some of those toys at over $7,000.00.

Cracker Jack have been around since 1871, when two Chicago brothers, F.W. and Louis Rueckheim were making and selling popcorn. They had a pretty good business and decided to add a bit of a twist to the run-of-the-mill popcorn. They added molasses and peanuts to the popcorn and sold it at the 1892 Chicago World's Fair, also known as the World's Columbian Exposition.

It was a huge hit but didn't have a name. However, in 1896 a salesman was munching on their popular popcorn, molasses and peanut combination and exclaimed, "That's a cracker jack!" And there you have it...the box of Cracker Jack became one of the most popular snack foods ever invented. If you stacked all of the Cracker Jack boxes that have been sold on end, they would reach around the earth 63 times. And one last tidbit: there are nine peanuts per ounce of Cracker Jack.

Croissants. The bakers in Vienna, Austria created the crescent-shaped pastry in 1683 to commemorate the city's successful stand against the army of Ottoman Turks in that year. The shape of the croissant is derived from the crescent emblem on the Turkish flag, and when the Viennese devoured the pastry, it symbolized Austria "swallowing up" the invading Ottoman army. Croissants made their way to France and became a major part of their petite déjeuner (breakfast). Croissants arrived in the United States during the 1920s, much to the delight of the average American.

Devouring croissants should not become a habit in this day and age. The nutritive value of a croissant is minimal, to say the least. A small croissant is 100 calories and 50% of those calories are from fat.

Cruciferous vegetables. The cruciferous vegetables are named for their cross-shaped flowers. This health conscientious family of vegetables contains bok choy, broccoli, Brussels sprouts, cabbage, cauliflower, collards, kale, kohlrabi, mustard greens, radishes, rutabagas, and turnips. They are considered to be the big guns when it comes to disease-fighting properties.

Broccoli and cabbage have been studied the most. They contain various phytochemicals (phyto = plant) including indoles and isothiocyanates. The isothiocyanates stimulate liver enzymes that detoxify carcinogens (cancer-causing substances) and they suppress tumor development in cells that have already taken certain steps toward developing a malignant tumor. Indoles detoxify carcinogens as well but they also alter estrogen metabolism. The indoles convert the most potent of all endogenous estrogens, estradiol, into the least potent forms, including estrone. The least potent forms do not have breast growth stimulating properties that estradiol has. So how about a Brussels sprout tonight to protect those breasts?

Cruciferous vegetables and cervical intraepithelial neoplasia. A small study presented at the March 1999 meeting of the Society of Gynecologic Oncologists suggests that the indoles, the phytochemicals found in cruciferous vegetables, may play a role in *reversing* cervical dysplasia, also referred to as cervical intraepithelial neoplasia or CIN. Twenty-seven women with CIN were given either a supplement of indole-3-carbinol (13C) at a dosage of 200-400 mg/day, or a placebo. By the end of the three-month study, half of the women taking the 13C supplements experienced *complete* regression of the condition, while none of the women in the placebo group did. One third of a head of cabbage contains 400 mg of 13C, however, this supplement is also available in pill form in health food stores in the U.S.

A brief digression—the Pap smear (Pap is an abbreviated term for George Papanicolaou, the last name of the physician who discovered the procedure). The average sexually active American woman endured the annual ritual of having a Pap smear. Without going into all of the details of the actual procedure, suffice it to say that the end result is the examination of cells removed from the outer layer of the cervix and endocervical canal. When the cytologist (the individual trained to examine the cytos, or cells) peers into the microscope, the cells stare back. The cells are described according to various sizes, shapes, and amounts. Of course, the goal is to have a completely normal-appearing Pap smear with all of the cells smiling sweetly back at the cytologist.

However, certain changes occur with infections such as the Human Papilloma Virus (types 16 and 18) that can gradually progress to cancer. Those changes occur over time, but the cell numbers, sizes and shapes provide clues. The terms used to describe the cellular changes include hyperplasia (too many cells), metaplasia (a cell that doesn't belong in that particular area of the body), and dysplasia (cells with abnormal shapes and sizes). Of the three cellular descriptions, dysplasia is the most ominous in terms of the likelihood of progressing to cervical cancer. So…back to the original story.

C
55

It appears as if a little cauliflower goes a long way in protecting your cervix from cancerous changes.

"Cauliflower is nothing but a cabbage with a college education."
—Mark Twain (1835-1910)

Curry. This popular Indian spice was named after a British general, Sir George Curry (1826-1890) stationed in India who was extremely fond of highly spiced foods.

Cutting boards—wood or plastic? Plastic. Plastic boards are dishwasher safe and easy to clean. They don't need the oiling that wood boards need and they come in numerous sizes, shapes, weights, and colors to fit your kitchen needs. It is recommended that you have at least two cutting boards, one for meats and chicken, and the other one for everything else. *Cook's Illustrated* magazine actually suggests having three cutting boards available at all times, with the third one for garlic and onions. Soft plastic and wood cutting boards can retain the smell of garlic and onions, hence the suggestion to have a third board for the odiferous members of the onion family.

Two highly recommended cutting boards from *Cook's Illustrated* include:
    Joyce Chen's Spot n' Chop Cutting Board $14.99 (polyethylene)
    Bemis' Dishwasher Safe Wood Large Utility Board $13.99 (wood Composite/ phenolic resin natural hardwood)
    You will notice that the second highly recommended cutting board is actually wood. It is dishwasher safe and doesn't warp when placed in the dishwasher. The top and bottom surfaces are wood veneer and the sides are covered with a waterproof coating.

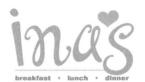
breakfast · lunch · dinner

Chickpea Dip
Makes 2 cups

1-1/2 cups chickpea (garbanzos) – canned
   3 cloves garlic – peeled
   3 Tbsp. tahini (sesame paste)
   6 Tbsp. water
   3 Tbsp. lemon or lime juice – fresh
   1 Tbsp. parsley – stems removed

Place all the ingredients in a food processor or blender and process until smooth.

Nutritional Info: For 1/2 cup serving: Calories 178; Total fat 8 gr.; Protein 8 gr.; Carbohydrates 21 gr.; Fiber 4 gr.; Sodium 11 mg.

D

is for...

Diabetes and
Dr. Pepper

Diabetes ("to siphon") Mellitus ("sweet").

"Taste thy patient's urine, if it be sweet like honey, he will waste away, grow weak, fall into sleep and die." —Dr. Thomas Willis

One thousand seven hundred new cases of type 2 diabetes are diagnosed in the United States on a daily basis. Type 2 diabetes is characterized by the body's inability to utilize insulin, the hormone that moves glucose, fats, and proteins into the cells to be used for metabolism. One of the reasons that the body has a hard time using insulin (also known as insulin resistance) is that it has *too much* adipose tissue. Adipose tissue is a fancy way of saying fat tissue.

Maintaining a healthy weight is absolutely critical when treating and/or preventing diabetes. Since excess adipose tissue is a major reason that the body cannot utilize the insulin produced by the pancreas, the simplest solution would be to lose weight. Easier said than done, I know, however, losing as little as 5-10% of your total body weight can reduce circulating blood glucose and can often avert the need for pills or insulin to control the blood glucose.

So just what is a diabetic diet? Or is there such a thing in this day and age? Standardized diabetic diets are out, individualized diet plans are in. The first step that should be made in controlling blood sugar is to consult with a registered dietician. She/he will explain that there are fewer dietary restrictions than previously used in the "diabetic diet." Diabetics should get 10-20% of their total calories from protein and divide the remaining 80-90% of the calories between carbohydrates and fats. Restricting carbohydrates is more important than restricting fats. Carbohydrates send a *big* signal to the pancreas to put out as much insulin as possible. You might think that this is a good response; since it appears as if the body is having trouble using the insulin produced by the pancreas in the first place. This is not the case. By flooding the body with too much insulin, triggered by excess carbohydrates, you increase the fat deposition in adipose tissue and the pounds start piling on. So, what is the bottom line here? You still should have fats in your diet and approximately 30% of the total caloric intake per day should be fats. Of those fats, 10% should be from saturated sources, such as butter. So, consider having a diet with 20% protein, 30% fat, and 50% carbohydrates. When choosing carbohydrates, pack your diet with whole-grain breads, bran cereals, and fruits and vegetables. Have a cookie or ice cream on occasion, but don't overindulge. Remember that the major *key* to controlling weight in this day and age is restricting caloric intake. A calorie is a calorie is a calorie, no matter which way you look at it. So, divide your calories into the above percentages and you just might prevent diabetes or you might lose enough weight to be able to discontinue your diabetic drugs.

Diabetes, insulin resistance and ethnic variations. Reduced tissue sensitivity to insulin is a major component in the development of type 2 diabetes. High-fat diets have long been known to reduce insulin sensitivity and it has been assumed that low-fat diets would improve insulin sensitivity. However, a recent study showed that this is not necessarily true and it depends on the ethnic group studied. Low-fat diets improve insulin sensitivity by 20% in Caucasian women but only by 6% in African-American women. High fat diets reduced insulin sensitivity by 6% in both Caucasian and African-American women. One other difference concerned leptin levels. (Leptin is a chemical produced by fat cells in the body. It signals the brain and tells us to stop eating.) On the high-fat diet, leptin levels increased 14% in African-American women, whereas levels didn't change in Caucasian women.

Diabetes and sugar intake. Sugar is no longer a no-no for those with diabetes, however, there is new evidence that sugar may play a role in the *development* of diabetes. JE Manson, M.D., of the Harvard Medical School found that women who ate diets high in refined carbohydrates and low in fiber were two-and-a-half times more likely to develop type 2 diabetes, regardless of age, weight or family history. Yikes. *Pump* up that fiber. You may want to consume whole grains, bran cereals, bananas, beans, and more beans, and nix the ice cream, cake and cookies.

Diabetes and waist size. Well, ladies…as you read this section, pull out the cloth tape measure found in your sewing basket and measure your waist size. Compare it to the list below and you may want to determine what your next course of action might be.

The risk of diabetes is 2.5 times greater with a waist size of 30-31 inches. The risk of diabetes is 4 times greater with a waist size of 32-33 inches. The risk of diabetes is 4.5 times greater with a waist size of 34-35 inches. This risk of diabetes is 5.5 times greater with a waist size of 36-37 inches. The risk of diabetes is 6 times greater with a waist size of 38 inches or greater.

DASH (Dietary Approaches to Stop Hypertension). Chalk up another plus in the fruit and vegetable column. In the DASH study, scientists at six medical centers across the U.S. studied 459 hypertensive adults for eight weeks. The participants were divided into three groups. The control group ate the typical all-American diet—high in total fats and saturated fats, low in fruits, vegetables, legumes, and whole grains. A second group ate a similar high-fat diet, but rich in fruits and vegetables (9-10 servings per day). A third group ate an overall healthful diet—low in fat and high in fruits, vegetables, low-fat dairy foods (3 servings per day), and other low-fat protein sources. The two groups eating lots of fruits and vegetables demonstrated significant reductions in blood pressure within two weeks. The overall healthful diet (group #3) demonstrated dramatic reduction in blood pressure over the entire study. Blood pressure in this group dropped an average of 11.4 systolic points and 5.5 diastolic points. In fact, the blood pressure reductions observed in this group were equal to those observed with antihypertensive drug therapy. The findings were attributed to the abundance of magnesium, potassium, calcium and fiber found in the healthful diet. The bottom line—dietary changes that focus on whole foods rather than individual nutrients can lower blood pressure quickly and effectively without the numerous side effects of drugs. The DASH diet is defined as: 26% of the total calories from fat (with less than 10% saturated fat), an increase in low-fat dairy products, 10-11 servings of fruits and veggies per day, and less than 3,000 mg NaCl per day.

See Appendix A for an example of a 2,000 calorie DASH diet. To learn more about the DASH diet see Appendix B.

Update on the DASH diet: As a follow up to the 1997 DASH diet, researchers have examined the role of sodium restriction and the control of hypertension. All participants in the study received the DASH diet, however, subgroups received different amounts of sodium with the DASH diet. One group received 3.5 grams daily (high sodium), the second group received 2.3 grams daily (intermediate sodium), and the third group received 1.2 grams daily (low). Mean systolic pressures ranged from 133 mm Hg in the high sodium group to 124 mm Hg in the low sodium group.

These results are basically the icing on the cake as far as sodium and hypertension are concerned. Dietary sodium restriction *does* lower blood pressure significantly and should be a part of the diet in hypertensive patients. The problem is, most processed foods in this country are loaded with salt. (Sacks FM et al. "Effects on blood pressure of reduced dietary sodium and the dietary approaches to stop hypertension" *New England Journal of Medicine,* 2001 Jan 4; 344:3-10.)

"The secret of staying young is to live honestly, eat slowly, and lie about your age." —Lucille Ball

---

Dehydration. What are some of the usual causes of dehydration? Exercise, high altitudes, caffeine, alcohol, and hot weather can all cause dehydration. Even mild dehydration, defined as a 2% loss of body weight can adversely affect health and exercise performance. How do you know if you are dehydrated? The point at which most people begin to feel thirsty is when 1-2% of their body water has been lost due to dehydration. So the key is to drink *before* you're thirsty, don't wait until you feel thirsty.

Q. How can you tell when a camel is dehydrated?

A. The state of dehydration in camels can be determined by the shape of the hollow in their sides behind the ribs. Diagnosis by this hollow area is so accurate that nomads can tell how dehydrated a camel is within 10 liters.

A well-hydrated camel usually drinks 10-20 liters or more per minute with a maximum speed of 27 liters per minute. The camel gulps only 3-4 times when gulping 1 liter of water. The camel can drink as much as 100 liters after going several days without water. When a large quantity of water reaches the blood and tissues of camels, it is diluted to an extent that could not be tolerated by other mammals whose red blood cells would rupture in less hypotonic solutions. The red blood cells of camels can swell to 240% of their initial size without bursting. The turnover of water in a camel is also low—82 ml/kg per 24 hours for camels grazing in the summer. This is about half the rate of cattle grazing in the summer. The winter turnover of water in the camel is half that of the summer rate.(Gauthier-Pilters H, Dagg AI. *The Camel: It's evolution, ecology, behavior and relationship to man.* 1981. The University of Chicago Press, Chicago IL.)

Dehydration and fatigue. Fatigue is one of the early signs of mild dehydration, according to Susan Kleiner, in the *Journal of the American Dietetic*

Association, February 1999. Dr. Kleiner recommends drinking 9-12 cups of decaffeinated beverages daily with 5 of the 9-12 as water. Caffeine is a diuretic and will only assist in perking you up while drying you out. Hence, decaffeinated beverages are recommended.

DIETS

"Probably nothing in the world arouses more false hopes than the first four hours of a diet." —Dan Bennett

---

Diets and high school wrestlers. A survey of 2,532 Michigan high school wrestlers uncovered the most common methods of a quick weight loss used by these young athletes. Sixteen percent tried to spit the weight away every day, while 22% did so 1-4 days a week. Other wrestlers wore plastic or rubber suits, fasted for more than one day, restricted fluids, used diuretics, took laxatives and/or diet pills and binged and purged. Doesn't sound too healthy and certainly not too smart—spitting weight away? *Where did that come from?*

DIGOXIN

Digoxin (Lanoxicaps, Lanoxin) and food interactions. The pectins in apples may bind to digoxin and reduce the effectiveness of the drug. Advise patients to not eat apples at the same time they take their digoxin.

DIOXIN

Dioxin and other closely related, dreaded chemicals. The dreaded chemical group consists of dioxin, furans, and PCBs (polychlorinated biphenyls). All of the three contain nasty benzene rings and can enter into the nucleus of cells to wreak havoc on the genetic material. Chemical damage to DNA can result in birth defects, such as neural tube defects (spina bifida), and abnormal cellular proliferation, or cancer. In fact, the Environmental Protection Agency estimated that the cancer risk increases by one in 100 for the most dioxin-sensitive individuals. This risk of getting cancer is over and above the risk of cancer from all other causes. So, this is not just a one in a billion chance. The risk for the average American is one in 1,000, above and beyond the other risks for cancer in an individual.

Other known toxic effects of these dreaded chemicals include developmental delays in children, reproductive changes in the males possibly including a reduction in testicular size, lower testosterone levels, and reduced sperm counts. In women, dioxin has been linked to a possible increase in the risk of endometriosis and possibly infertility. Immune dysregulation may also occur in dioxin-exposed individuals. It may make kids less responsive to vaccines and it may also increase the risk for allergic symptoms in certain groups of individuals. There is also some evidence that it may increase the risk of autoimmune diseases such as systemic lupus erythematosus, also known as "lupus."

Dioxins, furans, and PCBs are released into the air via municipal waste incinerators, hospital incinerators, and electrical transformers. People can inhale the particles, however, this is not the major route of entry. These toxins settle on grazing land, in lakes, in ponds, in streams, and other bodies of water. The cattle eat the dioxin-laden grass, and the fish and shellfish ingest small particles of dioxin-laced sediment. Dioxin and friends concentrate in the fatty tissues. Dioxin-tainted grain is also fed to hogs and cattle.

Dioxin works its merry way up the food chain as humans consume fish, shellfish, beef and pork. The "fattier" the fish, beef or pork, the greater the concentration of dioxin contained within. Vegans, who eat no animal products, ingest the lowest levels of dioxin. In contrast, the followers of the Dr. Atkins' diet, which is full of meat and seafood, ingest the most.

More than 90% of the human exposure comes from fish, meat, poultry, and non-skim dairy products. Fattier fish have more toxins than leaner fish. Shellfish like lobsters are low in fat, but the dioxin is concentrated in that "green stuff" that is pulled out of the body of the lobster. (By the way, that "green stuff" is actually the liver and pancreas of the lobster, combined in one green, gooey mass—ick.) So, pregnant women dining on lobster should be especially aware of the dangers to the developing fetus, and should not even consider eating that gooey green stuff.

Freshwater fish contain the highest amounts of dioxin, furans, and PCBs with an average of 274 picograms per 4 ounces of fish. Marine shellfish and marine fish are next at 95 and 70 picograms respectively. Beef measures in at 33, pork at 26, eggs (2) at 13 and milk (1 cup) at 11. Choose your foods wisely. Be especially careful about seafood, especially if you are in the mood or the mode to get pregnant.

Most of the seafood consumed in the U.S. is marine or farm-raised freshwater fish, which have lower levels of dioxin than wild freshwater fish. Two of the most commonly eaten fish are Pollock—the white fish that ends up in most fish sticks and fried fish sandwiches—and tuna. Catfish is another very popular freshwater fish—served in voluminous amounts at your favorite "Red lobster for the seafood lover in you." The good news is that most catfish and trout are not the "wild" type, but are farm-raised and fed largely plant meal, which means that their dioxin levels are very low compared to the trout and catfish swimming in streams and in the mighty Mississippi. (*Nutrition Action Newsletter,* October 2000.)

Disliked foods. The most disliked foods in America: tofu, liver, yogurt, Brussels sprouts, lamb, and prunes.

Diverticulitis, diverticulosis, diverticular disease. It is estimated that symptomatic inflammation of the diverticula, referred to as diverticulitis, will develop in only 20% of the patients with diverticula. The terms diverticulosis and diverticular disease usually refer simply to the presence of uninflamed diverticula. Diverticulosis is extremely common in Western society, affecting approximately 5-10% of the population over 45 years of age and almost 80% of the population over 85 years of age.

What are diverticula? And how do they become "itised" or inflamed? Diverticula are defined as herniations (out pouchings) of the lining of the large bowel or colon at areas of weakening next to blood vessels that penetrate the wall of the colon. The cause of colonic diverticula is related primarily to two factors: increased pressure inside the lumen of the colon and weakening of the bowel wall. Diminished stool bulk from insufficient dietary fiber leads to a reduction in gastrointestinal transit time (a fancy way of saying that stool sits in the large bowel for way too long) and to elevated colonic pressure. Once diverticula are present, particles of undigested food become imbedded within them. The opening of the diverticula becomes blocked or obstructed and this sets the stage for inflammation and the overgrowth of normal colonic bacteria.

The treatment for acute diverticulitis is oral hydration consisting of a liquid diet and 7-10 days of a broad-spectrum antibiotic such as ciprofloxacin (Cipro) and metronidazole (Flagyl). Once the acute attack has resolved, the patient should be instructed to maintain a high fiber diet. Hospitalization may be necessary if patients are unable to tolerate oral hydration.

D

65

Dr. Pepper. Why did Dr. Pepper bottles have the numbers 10, 2, and 4 written on the sides? These are the times that a person's blood sugars are lowest and can therefore be "revived" by a sugar drink such as Dr. Pepper.

Drug interactions with food. The Food and Drug Administration (FDA) has recently teamed up with the National Consumers League to publish a list of foods people should avoid when taking common medications. The following are a few examples of food and drug interaction. For a comprehensive copy of "Food and Drug Interactions," call 1-800-639-8140.

Anticonvulsants such as carbamazepine (Tegretol, Epitol) and phenytoin (Dilantin) increase folic acid metabolism and decrease intestinal absorption of folic acid resulting in decreased folic acid levels. Anticonvulsants also increase the rate of vitamin D metabolism leading to decreased levels of vitamin D. Give supplements of both if clinical judgment warrants it.

Glucocorticoids such as cortisone, Prednisone and dexamethasone prescribed for long term administration result in calcium and vitamin D depletion with steroid-induced osteoporosis. Supplementation with calcium and vitamin D as well as a bisphosphonates (such as Fosamax) is necessary.

Isoniazid (INH, Laniazid) interferes with vitamin B6 metabolism. Patients receiving greater than 10 mg/kg/day of INH should be supplemented with 50-100 mg of pyridoxine (B6) per day.

D

66

Date Chutney
Makes 1 cup

ina's

breakfast • lunch • dinner

- 1 cup dates – pitted, chopped (about 15)
- 1/2 cup lemon juice, fresh
- 1/4 cup water
- 3 Tbsp. cilantro, fresh - stemmed, chopped
- 1 Tbsp. jalapeno - seeded and chopped
- 1/2 tsp.kosher salt

Combine all the ingredients in a blender or food processor and process until thick and smooth. Will keep refrigerated for 2 days.

Nutritional info: 1 Tablespoon serving: Calories 33; Total fat 0.1 gr.; Protein 0.3 gr.; Carbohydrates 8.9 gr.; Fiber 0.9 gr.; Sodium 74 mg.

is for...
Egg-cetera

Eggs—the incredible edible egg. Egg consumption is down 20% since 1940 and 40% since its high in 1945. There has been a modest increase since 1995. The average weekly egg consumption has fallen from 2.3 in 1986 to 1.6 in 1999 in males and from 2.8 in 1986 to 1.4 in 1999 in females. The average American consumes 243 eggs per year.

- Each egg yolk contains approximately 215 mg of dietary cholesterol, which is 71% of the recommended daily value of dietary cholesterol. By the way, eggs are graded by the size of their yolks and the thickness of the white, qualities that affect appearance but not nutritional values. The higher the grade, the thicker the yolk and the thicker the white will be when you cook the egg. So, buy Grade AA eggs if you want to cook them sunny side up, because Grade B eggs will look rather puny and anemic on the breakfast platter.

- The regular egg sizes (Jumbo, Extra Large, Large, Medium, Small) are determined by how much the eggs weigh per dozen.

- One ostrich egg will make 11½ omelets.

- Most hard-boiled eggs end up with off-center yolks. This is why deviled eggs have defied automation for all these years.

- Two proteins, lysozyme and ovotransferrin, found in the egg white, are responsible for inhibiting bacterial growth in the raw egg. When the eggshell is intact, the chick embryo is protected from nasty pathogens. However, if the shell is cracked, the enzymes become ineffective and the egg is highly susceptible to bacterial growth. Once the shell is removed, raw eggs should be consumed within two days. Two other ways to keep eggs safe from infection include storing eggs with the small end down and not washing the eggs prior to storing them in the refrigerator. When the eggs are stored with the small end down the yolk is completely submerged in the egg white. The egg white contains the natural antibacterial proteins that protect the yolk of a developing chick embryo in a fertilized egg. If you wash the eggs before storing them the water will make the eggshell more porous, allowing pathogens a perfect portal of entry.

- *Salmonella* loves eggs. In fact, *Salmonella* can slip through the pores of an intact shell, without providing a clue to the unsuspecting consumer that they have contaminated the egg. So, as a general rule of thumb, *never* eat or serve a dish or beverage made with raw fresh eggs. Cooking eggs to an internal temperature of 145° F destroys the *Salmonella*. Egg-milk dishes such as custards must be cooked to an internal temperature of 160° F.

- Speaking of pores…the eggshell has between 7,000 and 17,000 pores that helps it breathe. Odors can permeate the egg through the pores, allowing the egg to absorb the odors of the surrounding foods in the 'fridge. Keeping the eggs in their original carton prevents the evening leftover Chinese takeout moo goo gai pan from permeating your freshly scrambled breakfast eggs. So, when purchasing your new refrigerator, don't pay extra for an "egg tray." It's a waste of money because you don't want to remove your eggs from their original carton for their storage.

- Brown eggs or white eggs? The color of the egg's shell depends on the breed of the hen that laid the egg and has nothing at all to do with the nutritive value or the taste of the egg. (I beg to differ. I can tell a brown egg from a white egg in a taste-test, blindfolded, hands tied behind my back.)

- Beaten egg whites can be used as a facial mask to make your skin temporarily look smoother. The mask works because the egg proteins constrict as they dry on your face, pulling at the dried layer of cells on top of your skin. When you wash off the egg white, you also wash off some of these loose cells. You can also use egg whites as a rinse or shampoo. The protein in a beaten raw egg can temporarily make your hair look smoother and shinier by filling in the chinks and notches in the hair shaft.

- Eggs are one of the top 12 foods triggering allergic reactions.

- Vaccines grown in egg cultures or in chick embryos include the live-virus measles vaccine, live-virus mumps vaccine, and vaccines for influenza. This may trigger an allergic reaction in people with a history of anaphylactic reactions to eggs.

- For more egg-citing information concerning eggs see Appendix B.

Egg a day is A-OK (except for diabetics). According to a study in the April 21, 1999 issue of the *Journal of the American Medical Association* the average American without diabetes can consume one egg a day without

FACT: The French are the most serious when it comes to food. Who else would codify 295 ways to prepare eggs – not counting omelets! In fact, the 100 pleats in a French chef's tall white hat, *la toque blanch,* traditionally signifies the number of ways he/she must know how to prepare eggs in order to qualify as a member of the profession.

adverse effects on the heart. After adjusting for other clinical variables, the researchers concluded that there was no relationship between egg consumption and the risk for coronary artery disease or stroke events in the overall population. Among diabetics who eat more than one egg per day, however, the risk for cardiovascular events doubles among men and increases by 49% in women compared to those who eat less than one egg per week.

NOTE: These data provide reassurance that an egg a day is *not* dangerous for the average American. Diabetics, however, should be prudent in their egg consumption.

Ephedra for weight loss. Ephedra (ma huang) is a popular ingredient in weight-loss and energy supplements. The most well-known of the weight-loss supplements is Metabolife, however, others such as KAL DietMax and Natural Trim also contain ephedra. Some studies have claimed that ephedra is safe and effective when used as directed. A study by the Council for Responsible Nutrition concluded that ephedra was safe if the dose was limited to 90 mg divided into three doses. However, right behind that study was another study from the University of California at San Francisco. The study combined 140 reports of ephedra-related adverse effects and found problems ranging from hypertension to strokes, seizures and death. The biggest concern was the dose discrepancy. Nine of the most serious events occurred at doses between 12 and 36 milligrams a day, which obviously is much less than the 90 mg dose recommended by the Council of Responsible Nutrition.

E

69

Esophagus. It take 4-8 seconds for a bolus of food to move through the esophagus to the stomach. Peristalsis moves food rapidly through this 10-inch tube in order to arrive at the stomach.

"With the possible exception of diet modification, we know of no single intervention with greater promise than physical exercise to reduce the risk of virtually all chronic diseases simultaneously." (Booth FW, Gordon SE, Carlson CJ, Hamilton MT. "Waging war on modern chronic diseases: primary prevention through exercise biology." Journal of Applied Physiology. 88:774-787, 2000.)

Exercise before you eat? Eat before you exercise? Should you exercise before or after a meal to lose weight? It depends on whether you are skinny or fat. Lean individuals burn more calories when they exercise after a meal, however, obese individuals burn more calories when they exercise before a meal. The difference in the number of calories burned isn't astounding. Lean individuals burned 7 more calories after eating and obese individuals burned 19 more calories when they exercised before eating.

"Whenever I feel like exercise, I lie down until the feeling passes."
—Robert Maynard Hutchins (1899-1977), former president and chancellor of the University of Chicago, dean of the Yale Law School, and chairman of the board for the Encyclopedia Britannica.

Exercise, water and rectal cancer. A study from Taiwan found that men who drank the most water (a quart, or 4 cups at least in a 24 hour period) had a 92% lower risk of rectal cancer than those who consumed 1.5 cups or less. Men who exercised the most had an 83% lower risk of colon cancer compared with the most sedentary men. (*International Journal of Cancer*, August 1999)

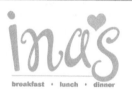

"The only reason I would take up jogging is so that I could hear heavy breathing again." — Erma Bombeck

---

Eggplant Dip
Middle Eastern Style
Makes 1¼ cups

ina's
breakfast • lunch • dinner

- 5 cups eggplant – 1" cubes, peeled (about 1-1/2 pounds)
- 1 cup red or yellow bell pepper – chopped
- 1 cup red onion – chopped
- 1 Tbsp. olive oil, extra virgin
- 2 cloves garlic
- 1 Tbsp. tomato paste
- 1/2 tsp. kosher salt
- fresh ground pepper to taste

Preheat the oven to 350 degrees. Line a cookie sheet with parchment paper or spray with cooking spray. Put the eggplant, pepper, onion and garlic on the sheet and coat with the olive oil.

Bake for 45 minutes until the vegetables are tender. Cool.

Place the vegetables in a food processor with the tomato paste, salt and pepper and process until smooth.

Nutritional info: Serving 2 Tablespoons: Calories 41; Total fat 1.8 gr.; Protein 1 gr.; Carbohydrates 6.2 gr.; Fiber 2.1 gr.; Sodium 121 mg.

F

is for...

Fear of Flatulence

"If we passed all of the gas we made, everybody would be farting a million times a day," sayeth the guru of gas passing, Dr. Michael Levitt, M.D. and GAS-troenterologist extraordinaire, Director of Research at the Minneapolis Veterans Affairs Medical Center. (By the way, the field of GAS-troenterology is not named after the odiferous emission known as flatus. It is from the Greek word, *gaster,* which means "belly.")

The average American intestine processes 10 liters of gas everyday. Ninety-nine percent of this gas is comprised of nitrogen, oxygen, carbon monoxide, hydrogen and methane. The nitrogen and oxygen come from swallowing air with meals and saliva. The typical swallow of saliva is accompanied by 15 ml of air. For people with a nervous habit of swallowing, that can add up to a significant bellyful of gas.

The zillions of bacteria found in your large intestine produce the other three gases—carbon monoxide, hydrogen, and methane. These bacteria are constantly champing at the bit for any morsel of food that sneaks past the small intestine. The food is fermented into gas, and, a heck of a lot of it—10 liters to be exact. However, we don't pass most of it (thank goodness), because a neighboring bacterium has the ability to consume it for personal use. If any gas is left over, it is expelled during a fit of laughter, a coughing spell, a contest amongst close friends, or just to impress the inebriated crowd that you're hanging out with.

For the record, the mean flatal frequency rate is 13.6 episodes per day with no statistical differences attributable to age, gender, or any other discernible variables. The upper limit for even the most gaseous among us is less than 25. The average person releases between 500 and 2,000 ml of gas per day via the rectum, with an average volume of 90 ml per expulsion for women and an average of 125 ml for men. Note the gender difference with this statistic—one that men are particularly proud of on any given expulsion.

The contents of the gaseous expulsion are generally rather benign. Hydrogen, nitrogen, oxygen and methane have little or no odor. However, the unpleasant fumes are derived from trace amounts of sulfur in the intestine—residue from meats and cruciferous vegetables such as broccoli, cauliflower, cabbage, and Brussels sprouts.

HISTORICAL HIGHLIGHT

In the early 1980s, colonoscopy procedures led to a few mini-explosions when stray electrical sparks reacted with intestinal hydrogen. These slight mishaps prompted gastroendoscopists to require that patients "fast" prior to undergoing the procedure. Of course, some enterprising physiology students learned of this side effect of hydrogen meeting an electrical spark. That, in turn "sparked" the late-night-fraternity-party-lighting-fart-frenzy to impress the partygoers.

What can be done about excess gas? Approximately 80% of the patients complaining of excessive flatus can benefit from dietary changes. Recognize the "gas triggers" such as the cruciferous family of veggies, as well as , onions, and hard-to-digest sugars such as lactose or fructose. These sugars are present in dietetic candies and sugar-free chewing gums. Also remember that chewing food thoroughly is better than gobbling and increasing water intake and exercise can improve digestion and reduce gas formation.

As a rule of thumb, the more carbohydrates you consume, the more gas you will produce. Vegetarians are usually *not* the life of the party, unless of course, they can perform the "lighted fart" trick popularized in the late 1980s. The switch from carnivore to vegan is particularly hazardous to your relationships—especially when the traditional diet is switched to one containing increased legumes and carbohydrates of various sizes and shapes. However, have patience. After two to four weeks the excessive passage of flatus will diminish and you can venture out in public once again.

People with lactose intolerance—trouble digesting milk or sugar, which can produce excessive gas—can be pinpointed with a breath test in the physician's office. In such cases, dietary alterations and taking lactase (Lactaid) may reduce gas, though it won't solve the problem completely.

Flatulence—treatment with over-the-counter and alternative medicines. Over-the-counter products include simethicone, the active ingredient in Gas-X and Mylanta Gas. Simethicone breaks up gas bubbles and makes them easier to pass.

Carminative herbs and spices include chamomile, mint, ginger, fennel, and crimin. Also, coriander and oregano are used to aid the digestion of foods that create gas. Plant-based enzymes including bromelain (from pineapple) and papain (from papaya) are available from health food stores for this purpose.

Certain cultures have traditional food additives that help keep flatulence in check. For example:

Indian preparations: A spice called *hing* is routinely used in bean dishes to reduce excessive passage of flatus.

Mexican preparations: Black beans are always cooked with *epazote*, another carminative herb.

Chinese preparations: *Fennel* has traditionally been used in Chinese dishes for cases of "excess wind."

Capsules of activated charcoal will absorb gas (and unfortunately anything else coming down the pike, so to speak, including vitamins, minerals, and medicines). Speaking of activated charcoal, you can purchase your own charcoal filter cushion known as the flatulence filter, formerly known as the Toot Trapper. This cushion lasts for 18 months, and absorbs up to 90% of the odor generated by a plate of pinto beans.

The makers of Beano have received a bit of support from the scientific community, as well as whole-hearted support from the teeming masses. The sample size of the initial Beano study was small, however, the results packed a powerful punch. Nineteen volunteers agreed to two lunches of cornbread, and meatless chili made with beans, broccoli, cabbage, cauliflower and onions. At the first lunch, one half of the volunteers consumed the chili, while the others were given a placebo made of water and Worcestershire sauce. A

HISTORICAL HIGHLIGHT

Consider the career of the French entertainer, Joseph Pujol. Born in Marseilles in 1857, his stage name was "Le Petomane" (Fr. to break wind). Pujuol mastered the anal sphincter abilities of voluntary inspiration, retention, and voluntary exhalation, so to speak. To inhale, anal sphincter relaxation was combined with reduction of intraabdominal pressure. He discovered that the tighter the sphincter during exhalation, the higher the pitch and the lower the timbre.

He became known as the man with the musical anus, and his performances at the Moulin Rouge thrilled audiences for 22 years. Bird trills, twitters, and warbles would precede an early version of the game that we now know as "Name that Tune." Requests were honored for various songs and jingles of the day, including "au Claire de lune." The range of a Pujol symphony could extend from a brassy blare to a "violinistic tremulo." The grand finale was to blow out a candle from a one-foot distance. His solo falsetto was such a hit that nurses had to revive the female portion of the audience. The ladies laughed so hysterically that they developed "corset-induced" hysterical syncope and passed out.

In 1781, Ben Franklin proposed that a scientific prize be awarded for the discovery of, "Some drug wholesome and not disagreeable, to be mixed with our common food, or sauces, that shall render the Natural Discharges of Wind from our bodies, not only inoffensive, but agreeable as perfumes."

week later, the volunteers and the lunches were reversed. A few drops of Beano accompanied all of the lunches. This was a double-blind study, so neither the volunteers nor the researchers knew when each diner would receive the real thing. Beano's function is to inhibit alpha galactosidase, the enzyme that breaks down sugars.

For six hours after each lunch the volunteers recorded the amount of abdominal pain, bloating and flatulence. Both groups reported the same amount of pain and bloating in the first four hours. The fifth hour was the clincher. The placebo group experienced almost four times the "flatulence events" of the Beano group—on average 1.9 events vs. 0.5 events per hour. One note: No one noticed a reduction in the smell factor.

Terry Graedon, a medical anthropologist and her husband, Joe, co-authors of *People's Pharmacy*, suggest keeping a "fart chart." In other words, keep a food diary and a chart showing when you pass gas. Remember that it's important to consider not only what you just ate for breakfast, but also what you had 8-12 hours earlier. For more information see Appendix B.

FAST-FOOD

Fast-food facts. Since the 1970s, fast-food restaurants have grown at a rate of 7% per year. The percentage of every American food dollar used for eating out has nearly doubled since that time, from 20%-38%. Portion sizes of restaurant meals, take-out foods, and snacks have also increased, in some cases by more than 100%. The number of restaurants that feature entrees with more than one portion size, e.g., "queen-size," "king-size," "super-size," "mega-size," has increased by 12% between 1988-1993. A typical bagel, once a skinny 2-3 ounces, has ballooned to twice that size, 4-7 ounces. The typical human has ballooned in the same way. Order any of the following at Chili's, Hard Rock Café, and TGIFriday's and this is what you'll get in return:

- Stuffed Baked Potato Skins: 79 grams of fat, 40 grams of which are saturated. Eight stuffed potato skins is equivalent to bombarding your heart with 2.5 pounds of Tater Tots.

- Buffalo Wings: 48 grams of fat, 16 of which are saturated. The average 12-wing order uses up 3/4 of your day's quota for total fat, saturated fat, and sodium.
- Chicken Caesar Salad with dressing: 46 grams of fat, 11 of which are saturated. The full-fat dressing is the culprit here. The croutons add a few grams of fat but watch the dressing.
- Bacon and Cheese Grilled Chicken Sandwich: 30 grams of fat, 12 of which are saturated. The bacon, cheese, and mayonnaise turn a heart-healthy grilled chicken sandwich into a heart attack between two buns. You would have to consume 8, count 'em, 8 McDonald's McGrilled Chicken sandwiches to get that much grease. Add French fries as a side order and the fat and sodium shoot up to your full day's quota...ouch...and the calories climb to 1,200...double ouch.
- Oriental Chicken Salad with dressing: 49 grams of fat, 12 of which are saturated. Like the Caesar, this salad has some semblance of health under all that gooey, fatty dressing. The skinless chicken breast sliced over lettuce, cabbage, carrots and other salad "stuff" is perfectly healthy. Keep the lid on that dressing. Also steer clear of the crunchy fried noodles that adorn the top or that accompany the salad on the side.
- Chicken fingers: 34 grams of fat, 13 of which are saturated. A typical five-finger order is as bad for your left main coronary artery as a Big Mac followed by a hot fudge Sunday. Yummy. So skip the chicken fingers and head straight to Mickey D's. How about if you add French fries to the chicken fingers? Oh, la,la...there goes the right main coronary artery and left circumflex. Don't forget the cole slaw and honey mustard dipping sauce and you're giving yourself one and a half days worth of fat, more than one day's worth of sodium and just over 1,600 calories. Ouch, ouch, ouch!
- Baby Back Ribs from Chili's: 54 grams of saturated fat, 21 of which are saturated. Add the French fries and cole slaw and you can turn your dinner into a Grand-Slam Denny's type double by-pass. Over 1,500 calories to fill those extra stretchy sweat pants with the elastic waistband.
- Mushroom burger with a side order of onion rings: You might as well just start planning your heart's funeral. This meal is the equivalent of 5 strips of bacon and four Dunkin' Donuts chocolate frosted doughnuts crumbled over three slices of Domino's Hand Tossed Pepperoni Pizza, slurped down with two Dairy Queen Banana Splits and a Big Mac. *This is not a good choice on any day, even a good day.*

F

75

Fats. Contrary to popular belief, fats are an essential component of the diet. Fats are necessary for proper growth and development of the brain and central nervous system. Fat provides essential fatty acids necessary for cell membrane structure and for prostaglandin formation. Fat also acts as a carrier for fat-soluble vitamins. Fat storage is important for energy production. So who said fat wasn't good for us? Perhaps he/she should have said, "Fat intake in *excess* quantities can be hazardous to your health."

An interesting paradox has occurred in the diets of the American public. The U.S. Department of Agriculture's Dietary Guidelines has stressed eating less fat and more carbs. So, the American public listened and started to watch their fat intake. However, something dreadful happened. We started getting even fatter and taking in more calories than ever, all the while, reducing *fat* intake. So, what was going on? Instead of eating high-fiber carbohydrates, the Americans decided to eat sweet, calorie-dense (translation: lots of calories in a small amount of food, like a box of low-fat cookies, low-fat cake, low-fat ice cream), low-fiber carbohydrates, so that the low-fat diet became a high-calorie, processed carbohydrate diet. And, the pounds started adding up. As a friend of mine once said: "Every time I go to Hannah's house to eat, she only has low-fat food. Low-fat this, low-fat that. Everything in Hannah's house is low-fat *except* Hannah."

Of course, the realization finally hit the government. *Calories do count.* Surprise, surprise. We also now realize that the type of fat is more important than the amount of fat. We now know that monosaturated fats and omega-3 fats are good for us, while the trans fats and saturated fats are bad for us. So, the diet can contain anywhere from 18% fat to 40% fat, depending on the type of fat and if calories are kept in line as well.

"Patience is one of the missing nutrients in most people's diets."
—Keith Ayoub, Ed.D, R.D. American Dietetic Association

Fat types. Good fats, bad fats, everywhere fat-fats. Low fats, high fats, some fats, no fats. Mono fats, trans fats, poly fats, sat fats, fish fats. So where do we start? How about from the really bad to the really good (in moderation of course)?

- **The really bad. The trans fats** form when vegetable oils have hydrogen molecules chemically *added* in the laboratory. The label of the product will say "hydrogenated or partially hydrogenated" but will not say "trans fats," although this is about to change due to new regulations from the government. Hydrogen molecules are added for specific reasons: 1) to make the fats solid at room temperature, 2) to make the product able to withstand frying temperatures, and 3) to extend the shelf life of products that use them as ingredients. Trans fats are abundant in stick margarines, shortening, pastries, packaged cookies and crackers, French fries, and other deep-fried fast foods.

Trans fats increase total cholesterol and the bad LDL cholesterol even more than saturated fats, the other bad guys. In very high amounts they may even decrease the good HDL cholesterol levels slightly. Any slight decrease in HDLs equals a big increase in heart disease. In fact, a 1-mg/dL decrease in HDL equates to a 2-3% increase in heart disease. In terms of heart disease, trans fats may be slightly worse than saturated fats, but suffice it to say, they are both bad for you. Recommendation: Minimal intake of trans fats. Looking at a pastry will supply you with all the trans fats you need for the day. The current intake of the average American is 2.5% of the total calories per day.

- **The bad. Saturated fats** are the "other" bad guys. Saturated means that their chemical structures are chains of fatty acids "saturated" with hydrogen molecules. That means that damaging oxygen molecules do not have a place to attach, making these fats less likely to be "oxidized" and become rancid. Saturated fats are abundant in animal foods such as meat, poultry (especially dark meat), butter, cheese, milk, and cream. They are also abundant in certain oils including coconut, palm, and palm kernel oils. There is *no doubt* in anyone's mind today that saturated fats, in abundance, contribute to heart disease, and possibly colon and prostate cancer. So "steer" clear, so to speak, of the saturated fats.

  So, how many saturated fats should the average American consume on a daily basis? No more than 8% of the total calories, which equates to 13 grams of saturated fat per 1,500 calories, or 18 grams per 2,000 calories. How is the average American doing with this recommendation? The current intake of saturated fats is *12%* of total calories. Looks like we have some work to do.

- **The sort of bad. Polyunsaturated fats** have chains of fatty acid with hydrogen bonds, however, there are two or more free areas for oxygen molecules to attach to. This means that they are susceptible to damaging oxidation. There are two types of polyunsaturated fats: the omega-6 and the omega-3.

  - ♦**Omega-6 fats.** The primary omega-6 fatty acid is linoleic acid, an essential fatty acid that the body cannot make on its own. Omega-6 fats are fairly heart friendly because they lower LDL and total cholesterol levels. Omega-6 fatty acids currently make up over 90% of the polyunsaturated fats in the average American's diet, mostly in the form of vegetable oil also known as seed oils. Soybean, corn, sunflower, and safflower oils are packed with omega-6 fatty acids. The problem is that too many omega-6s upset the balance between the 3s and the 6s. Corn oil, for example has a ratio of about 74 omega-6s to one omega-3. This is *not* good. The recommended ratio is less than 10 to 1 omega-6s to omega-3s. Too many omega-6s may also increase the risk of cancer.

  - ♦ **Omega-3 fats.** The other essential fatty acid, linolenic acid, (not to be confused with linoleic acid, and omega-6), is an omega-3 fatty acid. Studies have shown that omega-3s are good for you. They reduce clotting, prevent heart arrhythmias, boost immune function, promote eye and brain development, improve cognitive function and mood swings, and the list goes on. Most Americans do not consume enough omega-3s, hence the recommendation to bump up the weekly fish intake to at least twice if not thrice weekly. Fish oils are some of the richest sources of omege-3 fats, especially the fatty fish. Flaxseed oil is also a frontrunner in omega-3 fatty acids.

So then, how many polyunsaturated fats should we consume on a daily basis? Up to 10% of total calories (17 grams per 1,500 calories, or 22 grams per 2,000 calories), with more omega-3s and less omega 6s to reduce the omega-6 to omega-3 ratio to less than 10 to 1. Our current intake is 7% of total calories with a ratio of greater than 10 to 1.

• **The really good. Monosaturated fats** are the clear winner in the fat category. A mono fatty acid has one free spot (hence, the term "mono" or one), on its chain to which oxygen molecules bind. Two of the best sources are olive oil and canola oil; peanut oil and peanuts are high in monos as well. When monosaturated fats are substituted for saturated fats in the diet, cholesterol levels will improve. Mono fats may also offer some protection against breast cancer. Notice the word *may*. More research is needed to make a definitive statement but until that time it wouldn't hurt to increase the monosaturated fat intake while decreasing the polyunsaturated fats and saturated fats.

If you live in the Mediterranean countries your diet is traditionally comprised of 40% fat. However, the majority of the fats come from olive oil. Mediterraneans have a much lower incidence of heart disease, stroke and other chronic conditions due to their "good fat" intake.

Since this is the good stuff, how much should we consume? The recommendation is 12-20% of total calories as monosaturated fats, or 20-33 grams per 1,500 calories, or 27-44 grams per 2,000 calories. The current intake for the average American is 12-13% of the total calories. Here's an area that has room for a lot of improvement.

Fat content and food. Just how high is the fat content of that piece of chicken, slice of pizza or helping of Cheeseburger Hamburger Helper? Place the item on a paper napkin or paper towel and observe the grease mark. If it leaves an obvious grease mark, the item contains at least *3 grams* of fat. The greasier the spot, the greater the amount of fat. Here's the good news…keep blotting. It will help remove lots of those extra fat calories.

HISTORICAL HIGHLIGHT

If you have ever "chewed the fat," credit the crews of the old days of "wooden ships and iron men" who talked and grumbled while chewing their daily ration of brine-toughened salt pork.

F
78

Fat cells and gender differences. The fat cells of a 120-pound female can store an extra 74,000 calories; those from a 160-pound man can store an extra 95,000 calories. (Remember, 3,500 calories = 1 pound.) Women increase their body fat by 26% per decade of age, whereas men only increase their body fat content by 17% with each decade of age. Now, where is the Equal Rights Amendment (ERA) when we need it?

"Can you imagine a world without men? No crime and lots of happy fat women." —Nicole Hollander

---

Fat intake and migraine headaches. Reducing total daily fat intake to less than 20% of the total daily calories has been shown to reduce the frequency of migraine headaches by 70%, the intensity of the migraine by 68%, and the duration of the attack by 74%. (American Association for the Study of Headaches, Scientific Assembly, May 31-June 2, 1996, San Diego, CA.)

"No diet will remove all the fat from your body because the brain is entirely fat. Without a brain you might look good, but all you could do is run for public office." — Covert Bailey

FECES

Feces. The colon is home to more than 500 species of bacteria. Any given normal stool specimen may contain as many as 1,000,000,000,000 bacteria per gram of stool. Most of the nutrients from food have been absorbed on their journey through the GI tract. So a stool sample is 99% undigested fiber and the carcasses of billions of bacteria. Stool also contains a bit of potassium, however, not enough to cause a potassium imbalance unless the patient has copious amounts of diarrhea. And if they do, a potassium deficiency is not their only problem. An interesting corollary to this: when we have a patient with too much potassium (also known as hyperkalemia), we attempt to lower the potassium by giving enemas containing kayexelate and sorbitol. Both of these drugs assist in the removal of excess potassium by triggering peristalsis and diarrhea.

"If you need time to think, ask older patients to describe their bowel habits."
—Clifton Meador, M.D

FERTILITY

Fertility and dietary adjustments. Approximately one-quarter of women with fertility problems may be helped by dietary adjustments. Phytoestrogens (found in soy products, apples, carrots, and onions) may increase the length of the follicular phase of the menstrual cycle, resulting in fewer menstrual cycles over a lifetime. This translates into fewer eggs prepared for ovulation and fertilization. Women who have multiple risk factors for infertility may be more sensitive to subtle dietary influences. These women may want to avoid excessive intake of phytoestrogen-containing foods if they want to conceive. (*American Family Physician,* Quantum Sufficit, June 1996.)

FIBER

Fiber. When you hear, "Eat more fiber," just what exactly do "they" mean? Is there more than one type of fiber? Yes, there are actually two types of fiber, soluble and insoluble.

The insoluble fiber does not dissolve in water and basically goes right through you. This is the type of fiber that adds bulk to stool, causing it to push against the intestinal walls and move things right along. A good source of insoluble fiber is wheat bran. Whole grains, flaxseed, and the skins of many fruits and vegetables are other sources of insoluble fiber. When fiber is lacking from the diet, there's less stool, so the process of elimination slows to a crawl. When bulking up with that fiber, don't forget to add extra water as well. Water helps swell fiber, increasing its bulk.

The soluble fiber is referred to as water-soluble fiber and is the "sticky" fiber. It dissolves in water to a gel that binds cholesterol and removes it from the body. In other words, it takes excess cholesterol and transports it through the GI tract and out into the toilet. This prevents cholesterol from being reabsorbed back into the bloodstream and cholesterol levels are lowered. Soluble fiber comes from citrus fruits, dried kidney beans, psyllium, oat bran, apples, oats and barley.

So, soluble fiber for the heart? Insoluble fiber for the bowels? No one source of fiber is better than another source. Eat a variety of fruits, veggies, and grains totaling about 25 grams of fiber a day.

Flaxseed oil or ground flaxseed. Flaxseed has been used as food and medicine since ancient times. Hippocrates used it to relieve intestinal discomfort and it continues to be used for constipation and the pain of peptic ulcer disease today..

This nutty flavored seed is recognized as the best plant source of omega-3 fatty acids. It is also a great source of fiber and lignans, phytochemicals that help to prevent endocrine-related cancers including breast, endometrial, and possibly prostate cancer.

Flaxseed oil is not a good source for fiber, however the flaxseed is. It's about one-third soluble fiber, which accounts for its cholesterol lowering properties. The other two-thirds is insoluble fiber and accounts for its laxative benefits.

Grind the whole flaxseeds with a coffee grinder and sprinkle into cereal, yogurt, soups, and bread and pancake batters. If you mix the whole flaxseed into cereal, make sure you chew it well or the full benefit will not be recognized. Ground flaxseed can be refrigerated for 30 days without turning rancid.

More questions on flaxseed? See Appendix B.

F

81

Floaters vs. sinkers. One way to determine whether or not you have enough insoluble fiber in your diet is to observe the nature of the stool once it has made its final exit from your GI tract. Take a look at the stool (and don't tell me you don't look—*everybody* looks). If the stool is floating on top of the water (a "floater") in the toilet bowl, you can breathe a sigh of relief. You are consuming plenty of fiber in your diet. Stools float because of trapped gas from colonic fermentation of non-digestible fiber. If, however, the stool is torpedoing to the bottom of the toilet bowl (a "sinker"), you will need to bump up your fiber intake. It is recommended that we eat at least 25 grams to 30 grams of fiber per day in our diet.

Food-borne illnesses and older adults. Every day, about 200,000 Americans develop a food-borne illness. Of those, 900 are hospitalized and 14 die. According to the Centers for Disease Control and Prevention (CDC), about a quarter of the U.S. population suffers from food poisoning every year. Is this a new phenomenon? Yes, it appears to be. The CDC believes that the incidence of food poisoning has greatly increased during the past few decades. We eat more uncooked fruits and vegetables, which is great, however, if they are improperly grown or handled, they can easily transmit unhealthy pathogens. We eat more imported food, often from countries with lower safety standards than ours.

" In testimony before the Senate, it was suggested to us that food-borne illnesses may now be the largest reason for emergency room visitations by Americans. It is a virtual plague." —U.S. Senator Robert Torricelli (D-NJ)

And, our highly centralized and industrialized food-processing system has become an ideal means for quickly spreading newly emerged and dangerous pathogens such as *E.ColiO157:H7* and *Listeria monocytogenes* nationwide and around the world in less than eight days. When production-line workers try to keep up with the high-speed production line, they commonly make mistakes. Cow manure can be mixed with ground beef, and when ground into patties it can be widely distributed throughout the meat. Cow manure may be contaminated with *E.Coli O157:H7* and *Salmonella.*

The U.S. Department of Agriculture (USDA) tests hamburger meat for the National School Lunch Program in the U.S. In one 10-month period roughly 5 million pounds were rejected for contamination. Children are especially vulnerable to both pathogens and can develop a vicious diarrhea with both as well as renal failure with the *E.Coli O157:H7.*

One of the great ironies of our food safety program in the U.S., is that our food processing companies are centralized but the government agencies for food inspection are decentralized. More than one dozen federal agencies are responsible for inspecting our food. Here are some government facts that would be hilarious if they weren't so absurd. The Food and Drug Administration (FDA) regulates pizza, but if that pizza has hamburger, sausage or pepperoni as toppings, it falls under the jurisdiction of the USDA. The FDA regulates eggs, but chickens are regulated by the USDA. And, of course, we all know that any two government agencies have never seen eye to eye on anything, thus impeding efforts to reduce *Salmonella.*

The very young and the very old are prime candidates for food-borne illnesses, as are immunocompromised patients. Foods that are easily handled in our 30s, 40s, and 50s can be deadly in our 70s, 80s, and 90s. Our older population should consider a little more carefully whether the food they're eating could put them at risk for an infection from food-borne bacteria. In addition, immunocompromised groups such as transplant patients, cancer patients, and patients with HIV and AIDS should also be cautioned about the following foods:

Alfalfa sprouts, bean sprouts, radish sprouts and mung sprouts are all high on the list for developing food-borne illnesses from *Salmonella* and *E.ColiO157:H7*. The high level of moisture that sprouts need to grow provides the perfect environment for the pesky pathogens to persist and propagate. Since the sprouts are typically eaten raw, pathogens that can cause diarrhea, and something as serious as kidney failure don't get killed. Washing, even thoroughly, doesn't rid them of all of the pathogenic bacteria either. Fatal outbreaks of food-borne illness attributed to alfalfa sprouts have occurred not just in the U.S. but also in Japan, Finland, Norway, Australia, and Canada.

Deli meats and other ready-to-eat meats (hot dogs) and poultry products, smoked fish such as lox (smoked salmon) as well as refrigerated patés and meat spreads are perfect mediums for the culprit *Listeria monocytogenes*. Soft cheese such as feta, brie, camembert, blue-veined and Mexican-style varieties are also vulnerable to *Listeria*. Cooking can kill the culprit, but these foods are not generally heated at home after possible contamination at the processing plant. Symptoms of *Listeria* can range from gastrointestinal symptoms with cramping, nausea, vomiting, and diarrhea to life-threatening meningitis.

Caesar salad dressing, hollandaise sauce, eggnog, key lime pie (made with raw eggs) and any other dish made with unpasteurized raw eggs or undercooked chicken. In these foods the culprit is *Salmonella*. Raw unpasteurized eggs (as opposed to eggs in bottled Caesar salad dressing, for example) may contain *Salmonella* bacteria, which can bring on garden-variety GI upset such as nausea and diarrhea, but can also lead to serious complications such as severe dehydration. Runny and sunny-side-up eggs can contain *Salmonella* too. Eggs that are runny aren't exposed to enough heat to kill the bacteria that may be present, and the tops of sunny-side-ups never make it close enough to the heat source to kill any bacteria that may be lurking.

Approximately 2% of the juices sold in this country have not been pasteurized, meaning that it has not been treated to kill harmful bacteria, including *E.ColiO157:H7*. This bacteria causes an estimated 50,000 annual cases of food-borne illness, ranging from diarrhea and stomach cramps to renal failure and death.

Raw mollusks, including oysters, clams and mussels may be infected with *Vibrio vulnificus* or *vibrio parahaemolyticus*. Either of these bacteria can cause symptoms ranging from stomach cramps to fever to severe dehydration to bacteremia. People who may have low stomach acid (the case with three out of ten elderly people) are particularly vulnerable and should *never* eat raw mollusks.

F

83

Skip the salmon sushi if you want to enjoy raw fish at your local Japanese restaurant. Federal investigators tested fish in 32 Seattle-area sushi bars and found that servings of uncooked salmon (called *sake*) were infected one in ten times with roundworms that can cause illness in people. Raw tuna (called *maguro*), the most popular kind of sushi, wasn't a problem.

The high salt content of ham provides an ideal environment for *Staphylococcus aureus*. It multiples readily in ham left at room temperature. Cooking does *not* destroy the toxins produced by *Staphylococcus aureus* that make you ill.

Campylobacter jejuni **and food-borne illness.** The most common cause of food-borne illness in the U.S. is *not E.Coli O157:H7*, nor is it *Salmonella or Shigella*. It is none other than *Campylobacter jejuni*, the ubiquitous bacteria found in the intestines of poultry, turkeys and other birds. These bacteria are shed into "fowl feces" and proceed to cause misery in those who consume undercooked birds. Bloody diarrhea, fever, and abdominal pain are the most common symptoms. Approximately 4 million Americans acquire this food-borne pathogen every year in the United States. Deaths are relatively rare, between 200 and 1,000 per year, and mostly in the elderly or immunocompromised patients.

In about 1 per 1,000 cases, exposure to *Campylobacter jejuni* can trigger the development of Guillain-Barre syndrome, the demyelinating peripheral neuropathy that strips the longest nerves of their myelin. The patient experiences an ascending paralysis starting with the feet and moving up to the trunk and the muscles of respiration. Patients will usually recover, however full recovery depends on a number of factors. It is estimated that 40% of all Guillain-Barre cases are preceded by eating contaminated chicken one to three weeks prior to the symptoms. *Campylobacter jejuni* from undercooked chicken by one to three weeks.

Freezing the chicken will reduce the levels of *Campylobacter jejuni* contamination and cooking the poultry all of the way through will destroy it completely. *Campylobacter* does not multiply and spread rapidly and it cannot spread from one infected person to another. Most people who get *Campylobacteriosis*, as the infection is called, recover after about a week without treatment and without long-term sequelae.

Salmonella **and baby chicks—fighting flora with flora.** Preempt, a mixture containing the normal flora of the gut of healthy chickens, was approved by the FDA (1998) to spray on chicks as soon as they hatch. The mixture contains 29 benign bacterial species and helps prevent colonization of the chicks by *Salmonella*. It also has the potential to prevent *E. Coli O157:H7*, *Listeria*, and *Campylobacter jejuni*.

Salmonella has reached epidemic proportions in the U.S. It is responsible for two to four million cases of human illness per year. The Preempt mixture of healthy bacteria works by binding to all of the available sites in the intestines where *Salmonella* might otherwise bind. This strategy is known as "competitive exclusion."

This strategy basically mimics what mother hens naturally do for their baby chicks. The hens pass their own intestinal flora to their offspring when the young chicks peck at the mother chicken's fecal droppings. In our modern-day chicken-producing methods, baby hatchlings are separated from their mother hens at birth and are subsequently prevented from acquiring the normal maternal flora that prevents *Salmonella* binding. They are thus susceptible to colonization with pathogenic bacteria flora. (Stephenson J. "Fighting flora with flora: FDA approves an anti-*Salmonella* spray for chickens." *Journal of the American Medical Association*. 1998: 279; 1152.)

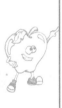

FACT: Pound for pound, chicken is 200 times more likely to cause illness than seafood (except shellfish) and 100 times more likely to result in death from that food-borne illness. When shellfish are factored in the numbers change. Raw and undercooked shellfish are 100 times more likely to cause illness than chicken and 250 times more likely to result in death.

F
85

FOOD PYRAMID

Food pyramid. The key to a healthy diet is to eat something from each of the most healthful five food groups every day: lots of whole grains, fruits and vegetables, low-fat dairy foods, and lean meat. All of the five groups are important. The top of the pyramid is *not* where you are supposed to start. It's the fats and sweets part and should be used sparingly. To see how your own diet compares to the recommended diet, add the number of healthy foods you eat from all of the pyramid categories except fats and sweets. Aim for at least 14 per day, with the ultimate goal of 23 per day.

If you would like to find out how to evaluate your own diet, see Appendix B.

As a reminder when you eat out, most restaurants turn the food pyramid upside down. The restaurant foods are heavy on the proteins, fats, and sweets and light on the fruits, vegetables and whole grains. Armed with that tasty tidbit, go through a mental checklist when ordering your meal. Grains?

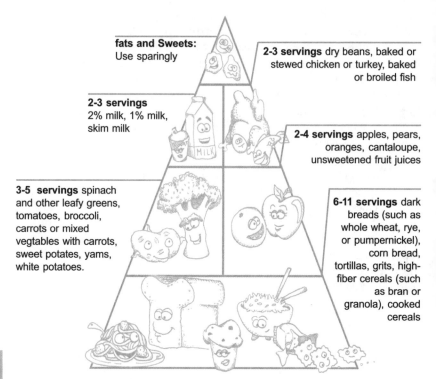

Fiber? Veggies? Fruit? How big is the meat portion? Two slices of pizza or the whole pizza? Thin crust or deep crust? Think thin, as in thin crust.

French fries. Gotta have 'em? Then choose wisely. Here's a list to take with you to the next fast food restaurant.

- McDonald's French Fries, small—2.4 ounces with 10 grams of fat, 210 calories, and 135 milligrams of sodium.
- McDonald's French Fries, *super-size* thighs, oops, I mean fries—7.1 ounces with 29 grams of fat, 4.5 of which are saturated, 610 calories, and 390 milligrams of sodium. Ouch.
- Burger King French Fries, small—2.6 ounces with 11 grams of fat, 230 calories, and 520 milligrams of sodium.
- Burger King King Size Fries packs 590 calories and 30 grams of fat, 12 of them saturated, and an eye-opening, jaw-dropping 1,100 mg of sodium.
- Hardee's French Fries (regular) and Jack in the Box French Fries (regular) are neck and neck in the categories of ounces (4), calories (340-

350), and fat grams (16). However, Jack in the Box wins the sodium war hands down with 710 milligrams of sodium versus only 390 milligrams for Hardee's. The clear winner (actually loser) for the sodium wars is Arby's Curly Fries, measuring in at 910 milligrams of sodium for a 3.8-ounce (small) order.

Frogs legs. A British slur on the French, referring to their penchant for the gastronomic delicacy of frogs' legs.

Frozen vs. fresh. Did you know that frozen fruits and vegetables are sometimes more nutritious than fresh fruits and vegetables? Frozen green beans contain twice the vitamin C as fresh ones that have been sitting for nearly a week on store shelves. Frozen and canned blueberries are just as nutritious as fresh blueberries. Blueberry growers freeze and can berries as soon as they are picked, which allows the berries to retain their antioxidant properties.

F

87

"A fruit is a vegetable with looks and money. Plus, if you let fruit rot, it turns into wine, something that Brussels sprouts never do." —PJ O'Rourke

The top 10 fruits that pack the most powerful punch. Tropical fruits are the clear winners in this contest. Paul LaChance, Ph.D., professor of Nutrition and Food Science at Rutgers University in New Brunswick, New Jersey, analyzed 31 popular fruits for 8 vitamins and minerals—vitamin A, Thiamin (B1), Riboflavin (B2), niacin, folate, vitamin C, calcium, and iron. *And the top winners are:* guava, kiwifruit, papaya, cantaloupe, srawberries, mango, lemon, orange, passion fruit, and red currant.
Coming in a close second: Raspberries and pears are full of fiber; apricots and bananas have loads of potas-

sium, and apples are rich in flavonoids (plant chemicals that help protect the normal growth and differentiation of cells).

"Avoid fruits and nuts. You are what you eat." —Jim Davis

FUDGE

Fudge. According to the *Oxford English Dictionary*, the first definition of the word "fudge" was "nonsense or foolishness." A candy-maker in Philadelphia was supervising his employees as they made caramels. Someone on the caramel line was having a bad day and instead of producing a chewy candy, the batch of caramels turned into a finely crystallized, nonchewy substance. The candy-maker screamed, "FUDGE!" and now you know the rest of the story.

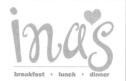

breakfast • lunch • dinner

Fruit Ambrosia
Serves 4

1	16 oz. can pineapple - chunks in water, drained
2	cups yogurt - vanilla non-fat
1/4	cups dried cranberries, blueberries or cherries
2	oranges (or tangerines), small - peeled, sectioned and seeded

Combine all the ingredients into a medium bowl. Cover and chill.

Nutritional info: 1 serving: Calories 239; Total fat 4 gr.; Protein 7 gr.; Carbohydrates 42 gr.; Fiber 3 gr.; Sodium 75 mg.

is for...
Garlic, GERD, and Girdles

Garlic *(Allium sativum)*. Garlic is a member of the onion family and has been used for medicinal purposes since the earliest recorded history of food and medicine. In the Egyptian writings of 1500 B.C., garlic was reported to have 22 medicinal uses, including the use for the prevention of heart disease, the treatment of headaches, and the prevention of fatigue. The Greeks used garlic to protect the construction workers who built their pyramids. The literature doesn't discuss what garlic protected the workers from, only that they were protected when they consumed the clove of the garlic. Roman soldiers consumed garlic on long marches to boost their energy and endurance levels. Louis Pasteur identified its antiseptic properties in 1858. During World War II, garlic was used as a salve on wounds for its purported bactericidal effects.

Garlic contains more than 100 different sulfur compounds. The compound associated with its healing powers and unfortunately its odoriferous powers is allicin. This compound is produced from allicin when garlic is crushed, cut, chopped, crunched or munched. Garlic powder also retains the medicinal allicin, as does cooked garlic. It appears as if allicin blocks certain enzymes associated with bacterial, fungal, and viral infections (Weitzmann Institute in Israel). Garlic's major vitamin contribution to the world of nutrition is vitamin C and its major mineral contribution is potassium. Central California produces more garlic than any other state or country—an average of 250 million pounds per year. And, the garlic capital of the world is Gilroy, California, a 90-minute drive south of San Francisco. For more information on Gilroy, see Appendix B.

Garlic's nickname is the "The Stinking Rose." The name is derived from a British Social Club where patrons munched on garlic as they sipped on their favorite adult beverage.

Garlic and bleeding time. Is there such a thing as a garlic overdose? Perhaps to friends in your immediate environment there is, but basically the answer is no. One important point to remember—garlic inhibits the clumping activity of platelets. If platelets fail to aggregate or clump, one can experience a prolonged bleeding time. (The normal bleeding time is 3-6 minutes.) This would only be medically relevant if the individual is also on other platelet-inhibiting drugs such as aspirin, ibuprofen, or an anticoagulant such as warfarin (Coumadin).

Garlic and colon cancer prevention. "Six cloves a week, keeps your bowel at its peak." Take it in raw or cooked form, but not supplements for colon cancer protection. (*American Journal of Clinical Nutrition*, October 2000)

Garlic breath. When you cut into a garlic clove, you tear its cell walls, releasing an enzyme that converts sulfur compounds in the garlic into ammonia, pyruvic acid, and diallyl disulfide. Diallyl disulfide is excreted in perspiration and in the air you exhale, which is why eating garlic makes you smell garlicky.

Garlic, natural or supplements? The majority of studies on garlic's health benefits have been performed with garlic powder supplements. Supplements are not only more convenient for the average American, they are most likely safer as well. Processing the garlic into the powder form removes any microbial contamination that may have been picked up in the soil (e.g., *Clostridium botulinum*). If the garlic tablet is enteric-coated it bypasses the stomach for metabolism, and it has more of a chance to be odor-free.

The usual recommended dose for natural garlic is one to two cloves a day. This equates to one large clove or two small cloves. The usual recommended dose for supplementation is 600-900 mg, divided into two to three doses per day. Supplements should contain the recommended standardized dose containing 1.3% of the active ingredient allicin, which provides the equivalent of approximately one fresh clove daily.

The caveat here is that many "fly-by-night" dietary supplement companies conveniently fail to add the active ingredient or they add such a small dose of the active ingredient that it does not provide one iota of health benefits. In fact, in one study of garlic supplements, 93% of the so-called standardized products were lacking sufficient amounts of allicin.

Garlic, raw or cooked? A plethora of controversy surrounds this $64,000 question. Most experts agree to disagree as to whether cooked or raw provides the most benefits. Literature from The Garlic Information Center states that cooked garlic still retains many of its active compounds and therefore, cooked garlic is still beneficial for health. One benefit of cooked garlic that no one denies—cooking can reduce the fairly annoying side effects and the pungent odor of raw garlic.

Cancer-fighting compounds that decompose on heating are called the allyl sulfides. That's why most experts advise that garlic be eaten in its raw form or in pill form to get the cancer protection benefits of garlic. Scientists at Penn State University have found a way to preserve the allyl sulfides during cooking. After chopping the garlic, let the garlic sit for at least 10 minutes prior to cooking. Having it sit for this period of time sets off a chemical chain reaction that dramatically boosts levels of the cancer-fighting allyl sulfides, allowing it to maintain its effectiveness when baked, sautéed, or microwaved.

Garlic supplements and cholesterol. In an October 2000 report, the Agency for Healthcare Research and Quality (AHRQ) of the U.S. Department of Health and Human Services found that garlic supplements did not lower cholesterol for long enough periods to improve health, yet manufacturers of popular garlic supplements such as Kwai, One A Day, Nature Made and Centrum Herbals, claim that they do.

AHRQ evaluated 37 randomized trials that tested the effects of garlic supplements on cholesterol levels. Small reductions occurred when patients took garlic for one to three months, but not when they took it for six months or longer. Prolonged elevations of cholesterol promote vascular disease; therefore garlic supplements are useless in preventing the disease over time. NOTE: This report only studied garlic *supplements*, not fresh garlic.

Garlic supplements and HIV protease inhibitors. Garlic supplements can interact with the protease inhibitors used in many treatment regimens for patients with HIV (Human Immunodeficiency Virus). Many HIV+ patients are using garlic because of its purported benefits as an antiviral and immune-boosting supplement. In addition, garlic has been shown to temporarily lower total cholesterol levels and to reduce triglycerides—both of which can be elevated with protease inhibitor therapy.

A new study shows that garlic can lower the serum levels of the protease inhibitor saquinavir (Fortovase, Invirase) by approximately 50%. Researchers suspect that a substance in garlic speeds up cytochrome P450 (3A4) enzymes that metabolize saquinavir and other protease inhibitors such as aprenavir (Agenerase), indinavir (Crixivan), ritonavir (Norvir), and nefinavir (Viracept).

Garlic might also affect other antiretrovirals that are metabolized by this enzyme system found in the small intestine. These include delavirdine (Rescriptor), efavirenz (Sustiva), and nevirapine (Virammune).

Ask HIV patients if they are taking garlic supplements. Garlic found in food is not likely to cause the same problems. To be on the safe side, advise HIV patients to avoid consuming more than one clove of garlic per day on a regular basis. (Piscitelli SC, Burstein AH, Welden N, et al. "Garlic supplements decrease saquinavir plasma concentrations." 8th Conference on Retroviruses and Opportunistic Infections, Chicago Illinois, February 2001.)

Garlic supplements and other drugs. Also watch for transplant patients who might be taking garlic along with cyclosporine (Neoral,

Sandimmune). Reduced cyclosporine levels in these patients may cause transplant rejection. Women taking oral contraceptives while taking garlic supplements should use another form of birth control to avoid unwanted pregnancy. (Jellin JM, Gregory PJ, Butz R, et al. *Natural Medicines Comprehensive Database.* Stockton California: Therapeutic Research Faculty, 2001.)

Garlic, vampires and werewolves. Vampires and werewolves may have a physiologic basis. A Canadian chemist has correlated the appearance and actions of vampires and werewolves with an extreme form of the disease known as porphyria, an inherited red blood cell metabolic disorder. Individuals with porphyria appear to have paws instead of hands and their lips and gums are so taut that their teeth become very prominent and fang-like. In the most severe cases, their teeth and bones will fluoresce in reaction to light. Their skin is hypersensitive to sunlight (hence, they abhor sunlight as vampires of lore traditionally did).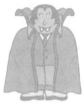

All porphyrias have as their root cause a lack of a specific enzyme required in the making of heme, the iron-compound responsible for making blood cells red and for the oxygen carrying capacity of hemoglobin. The cells in most porphyria patients can produce heme, but are only able to make a certain amount. Since taking heme in any form (sucking blood for instance) turns off the heme pathway this may treat one of the symptoms that patients complain about—severe abdominal pain. Since intravenous infusions of blood were not available in the Middle Ages, the next best thing was to drink a pint or so of blood.

Victims suffering from porphyria also react adversely to the chemical allyl disulfide in garlic—reputed in folklore to ward off werewolves and vampires. For sensitive porphyria patients, garlic may precipitate an attack. It is this link between garlic and porphyria that is considered to be the strongest proof that Count Dracula suffered from porphyria. Legend has it that Dracula and other vampires shied away from garlic.

In Wakefield, RI, citizens are banned from entering a movie theater within four hours after eating garlic.

GAS STOVES

Gas stoves and asthma. Women who cook on gas stoves have 2.5 times more asthma than women who cook on electric stoves. In addition, these women have twice the normal risk of wheezing, breathlessness, and waking up at night with shortness of breath. Nitrogen dioxide is the most likely culprit. It is a known bronchospastic agent and is also found in the smoke of wood-burning stoves and secondhand smoke.

Gastroesophageal reflux disease (GERD). There is a physiological sphincter between the esophagus and the stomach. In other words, a muscle tightens the sphincter in order to keep acid from the stomach backing up (known as reflux) into the lower one-third of the esophagus. When acid reflux occurs, the individual will complain of a burning sensation under the sternum. The old name for this burning sensation was heartburn; the new name is gastroesophageal reflux disease, or GERD. Risk factors include the consumption of certain foods and beverages (fatty or highly acidic foods, caffeine, chocolate, alcohol, spicy foods, and tomato products), especially within 3 hours of reclining for the evening , body position (reclining, bending over), stress, smoking, obesity, and certain medications (nitroglycerine, beta-agonists for asthma, calcium channel blockers.) So, how about a big, spicy Mexican dinner accompanied by a couple of shots of Tequila, followed by a chocolate éclair, cup of coffee and a cigarette? What are the chances of developing heartburn, or GERD, after that extravaganza?

Gastroesophageal reflux disease (GERD) and "alarm" symptoms. Three symptoms that indicate possible serious disease in patients with chronic GERD are: difficult or painful swallowing, hoarseness, and wheezing. Patients with any of these alarm symptoms need further evaluation for GI problems such as hiatal hernia, erosive esophagitis, diffuse esophageal spasm, and peptic ulcer disease.

Gastroesophageal reflux disease and sleeping on the left side. In addition to chewing gum (see the end of this chapter), tell your patients to snooze on their left side when napping. It appears as if GERD is more pronounced in individuals who sleep on their right side, so logically, one should roll over and try the left side. Gastric acid takes longer to clear from the esophagus of right-sided sleepers compared with those who sleep on their left side, back or stomach. The lower esophagus bends to the left, and when sleeping on the left side gravity straightens out the curve, making it easier for acid to flow out of the esophagus. Advise your patients to sleep on their left side and to use a pillow behind the back to maintain this position.

GERD capital of the world. According to *American Demographics*, Birmingham, Alabama wins this prize, with 72% of the adult population of this city claiming to have heartburn. The number two spot is held by Tucson, Arizona, with 62% of adults complaining of problems with heartburn. Rounding out the top five are Minneapolis (60.5%), Miami (60%) and San Diego (60%).

Gender differences and favorite foods. When asked to name their favorite foods, obese men answered "steak and roasts." Obese women responded with "doughnuts, cookies and cakes." The second favorite meal for obese men was ice cream and frozen desserts, however, obese women chose bread, rolls, and crackers. Third on the list for men was chicken and turkey, and the women preferred ice cream and frozen desserts as their third choice

"Whoever could make two ears of corn or two blades of grass grow upon a spot of ground where only one grew before would deserve better of Mankind, and do more essential source for his country than the whole race of politicians put together."
The King of Brobdinghag, Gulliver's Travels by Jonathan Swift, 1727

G
94

Genetically modified foods. The proponents of genetically modified foods (GMF) would certainly agree with The King on this one. And I don't mean Elvis. The benefits of genetically engineered plants include: insect resistance, herbicide resistance, virus resistance, delayed fruit ripening, altered oil contents, and pollen control. In other words, scientists can develop foods that resist disease, that can travel around the world without spoiling, and can provide more bang for the buck, so to speak.

The opponents of genetically modified food products refer to them as "Frankenfoods." They are concerned that the technology is not precise enough to avoid causing unwanted traits to be passed to a new plant form such as antibiotic resistance, or that it might cause health problems including allergies. They cite the October 2000 recall as a perfect example of what can happen with genetically modified foods. Taco shells containing the StarLink brand of corn were pulled from grocery shelves because the corn, developed for animal consumption, was not approved for human consumption. This corn had been genetically modified to produce a protein to kill crop-destroying caterpillars, and that protein had the potential to cause allergic reactions in humans.

So, what's all the fuss? What is a genetically modified food? Genetically modified foods are from plants that have had their genetic material altered in a way that produces new functions, using genes that come from many sources. We are all dining on genetically modified foods already. We have tomatoes designed to delay ripening. Potatoes, rice, papaya and squash have been genetically engineered to repel insects and resist disease. Many processed foods containing soybeans or corn have been grown from genetically modified seeds. In fact, more than half of the U.S. soybean crops grow from GM seeds and approximately 60-70% of packaged grocery products contain genetically modified organisms.

When genetically modifying a product, a small piece of an organism's genetic material or DNA, is inserted into another organism, transferring the desired trait. The plants and animals involved are not even genetically related. For example, a gene found in cold-water fish confers tolerance for cold. This makes sense. How else would a halibut live off the coast of Alaska without turning into a fish-sicle? In order survive it developed a gene that provides a type of "antifreeze" substance in the blood to prevent the fish from freezing.

Plant engineers have taken this concept one step further. They have removed this piece of genetic material from the cold water fish and inserted it into a tomato in order to make the tomato frost-resistant. Brilliant. Frost and freezing can destroy an entire crop of tomatoes. These GMF tomatoes have not hit the market yet, as they are still undergoing testing for safety concerns. Once they pass the test, we will be seeing frost-resistant tomatoes accompanying our meals.

As of January 2001 there are 12 genetically engineered plant species that have been approved for commercial production. These include corn, cotton, potato, tomato, soybeans, canola, sugar beets, rice, flax, squash/zucchini, papaya, and chicory. Genetically modified foods have found their way into nearly 4,000 food products, ranging from veggie burgers to ice cream, according to data from the Center for Plant Biotechnology Research at Tuskegee University in Alabama.

How do you know if the food you are consuming is genetically modified? You don't. The government does not require any special labeling for GM foods unless the food differs in safety, composition or nutritional quality compared to its natural counterparts. At this time, no food currently falls into this category.

Genetically modified foods as vaccines. In 1991 the World Health Organization challenged scientists to create a simpler, safer, cheaper way to vaccinate children. Scientists accepted the challenge. Syringes and needles are so expensive to developing countries, why not make an edible vaccine? Since plants produce a myriad of proteins, the scientists decided to attempt to engineer plants to produce specific proteins from a pathogen to stimulate the body's immune response.

The first plant considered for an edible vaccine was the potato plant. Potatoes grow in many areas around the world, they are cheap to grow and they are easy to store and ship. So the scientists inserted the gene from a specific protein from the cholera bacteria into the genes of the potato plant. The result was a genetically modified potato that stimulated the immune system. Stay tuned. Bananas are also on the list for use as an edible vaccine.

Genetically modified potatoes may also hit your local fast food restaurant in the near future as well. When a potato is fried, the oil that it is fried in replaces the water in the potato. Hence, French fries are harbingers of saturated fats. *But,* the starchier the potato, the less oil it soaks up and obviously the less fat consumed by the consumer. McDonald's pays a premium price for the 3.2 billion pounds of starchy potatoes it uses every year. Potatoes that are full of starch make crisper, less greasy fries. Scientists are attempting to develop potatoes with even *more* starch so they will soak up even less oil. To learn more about genetically modified foods see Appendix B.

GI (gastrointestinal) transit time. What is the GI transit time? It's a fancy way of explaining how long it takes food to travel from the mouth to the toilet. In humans, the residues of a high fiber, low fat meal typically make the big splash around 18 hours after the initial bite. The residues from a high fat, low fiber meal may not see the whites of a toilet bowl for 72 hours. Hummingbirds, on the other hand, have a GI transit time of less than one hour for the nectar to wind its way into the great hummingbird toilet in the sky. For the big snakes, transit times may be measured in days or weeks. It takes about 12-14 days to process a rat through the GI system of your basic rat-consuming python. Speaking of snakes:

Snakes, the digestive system. Humans consume small meals at regular intervals several times a day. In other words, our 16 feet of intestinal tubing is working most of the time and doesn't have to adapt to a very wide range of food intakes. This makes our intestine's responses modest in scope and difficult to study and analyze. Enter the anaconda, boa constrictor and the four python species of the Old World and Australia. These giant snakes are notorious for consuming humongous meals at long and unpredictable intervals. Since their meals are so massive, their intestinal responses must be equally huge, making these responses quite amenable to study as models of our own digestion.

The largest snake on record is a 37-foot anaconda. The longest snakes can be as thick as a man's waist and weigh several hundred pounds, most of it muscle. The muscles allow the snakes to squeeze their prey to death. The victims, interestingly enough, don't suffer broken bones and tend to retain their original shape while sliding through the snake's GI tract. Case in point: a 14-year-old Indonesian boy was swallowed by a reticulated python and his body was still intact and recognizable in the snake's stomach when the snake was killed and cut open two days later.

Swallowing a human being is not an everyday occurrence in the life of the reticulated python and there are only a few authenticated cases. You can breathe a sigh of relief if you are of the male gender and an adult—all cases have been small children or small women. These unfortunate individuals had to have been unconscious for some reason, as they would never have stood by idly while the snake devoured them for over an hour.

Do you remember how your mother used to admonish you for not chewing your food thoroughly? Well, snakes don't chew their food they just swallow it whole. The biggest prey on record is a 130-pound antelope swallowed by an African rock python. Another record-breaking case involved an Asian reticulated python gulping down a 28-pound goat and a 39-pound goat at one sitting. Two days later the same snake snarfed down a 71-pound ibex.

Are you impressed yet? How about a few comparisons in terms of relative body weights? Sheer gluttony in a human being may result in consuming a few pounds of food at one sitting, and 10 pounds would be practically unheard of. Even eating 10 pounds would be under 10% of our body weight. By comparison, a giant snake regularly consumes 20% of their unfed body weight and if particularly ravenous on any given day, it can easily eat 65-96% of their body weight. Let's open the Guinness Book of World Snake Records—a viper swallowed a lizard 1.6 times its body weight. What would that equate to in the Guinness Book of World Human Records you might ask? It would equate to a 140-pound male downing a 35-pound T-bone and occasionally swallowing a 224-pound side of beef.

So, if snakes only swallow foods whole, why bother having fangs? Snakes bite their prey but they don't chew it. The bite merely anchors the prey so that the prey cannot back out of the snake's mouth. Ugh. The fangs actually curve back toward the snake's stomach, so once the fangs engage it is virtually impossible to disengage.

The snake's jaws can open to an angle of 130 degrees, as compared to the human ability to open the jaw at a measly 30 degrees. In addition, the lower jawbone of the snake is hinged with two bones connected by a ligament. This allows for greater flexibility, which enables the snake's head to literally stretch around its prey.

One major problem with a huge meal is the time it takes to digest the food. The digestive process of the snake has to compete with the microbes of the GI tract of the digested victim. Dead animals begin to putrefy as their own bacteria begin to break down their bodies and release toxic chemicals. So, the bigger the victim is the greater the risk of a prey rotting in the snake's stomach.

This brings us to a simple explanation of why snakes enjoy basking on a rock out in the sun, and why they coil up to conserve heat. Heat speeds up the digestive process and reduces the probability of putrification of the devoured prey. An Indian python, fed a rabbit, completed digestion in 4-5 days when kept at a temperature of 82° F; however, when the temperature was reduced to 71° it took 7 days, and when the temperature was reduced to 64° it took 14 days. In fact, if the temperature gets too cool, the snake will refuse to eat anything at all.

The interval between swallowing and defecating may be quite lengthy (approximately 12-14 days for a rat), but the time between feedings may be even longer. Pregnant female rattlesnakes may go one and a half years without a meal. Zoo snakes have been known to refuse food for over two years. Snakes in the wild have feeding intervals of weeks to months. So the three square meals per day in the homo sapien population certainly doesn't apply to the snake population, nor does the daily, gotta' have it, bowel movement that obsesses a large proportion of the human population.

When a python swallows a mouse, its intestine doubles or triples in weight overnight. Each cell of the intestinal lining enlarges and produces longer finger-like villi to increase the surface area for digestion. By analogy, a 150-pound man would have to add six pounds to the weight of his intestine overnight. The snake has a 60-fold increase in the amount of enzymes produced for digestive purposes. In addition, it has a 3,600% increase in oxygen consumption as compared to the human's 20% increase in oxygen consumption after a meal. The cost of making extra intestine and digestive enzymes is so high that the snake uses approximately one-third of the energy it gets from the mouse's body just to consume the mouse. Wow.

Gin and tonic dermatitis. It's not the gin and it's not the tonic that causes that itchy rash. However, it's that oh-so-tasty lime squeeze that can trigger the sunburnlike dermatitis. This may be especially hazardous for your backyard bartender, since sunlight tends to trigger this photosensitivity reaction. Limes, celery, or parsnips are all culprits. What's with a gin and tonic with a twist of parsnip?

Ginger *(Zingiber officinale)*. Ginger has been used for medicinal purposes in China for more than 2,500 years. It is recommended for the treatment of dyspepsia, colic, flatulence, nausea/vomiting, fluid retention and motion sickness. The anti-emetic properties of ginger are thought to be through local action on the stomach mucosa, not through central brainstem mechanisms.

Gingivitis (inflammed gums). It takes 16-24 hours for the bacteria in the mouth to produce the plaque that contributes to gingivitis and peri-odontal disease. Therefore, brushing after every meal to prevent plaque is an unnecessary expenditure of time and energy. If you brush properly in the a.m. and p.m. and throw in one flossing episode with either, plaque problems will be history.

Ginkgo (*Gingko Biloba*). Gingko, also known as the Maidenhair Tree, is the oldest living tree species. Gingko trees have existed for over 200 million years. This herb is especially popular in Europe, where it is one of the most prescribed and lucrative of all herbal products.

Gingko has been shown to improve circulation by dilating the arteries as well as the veins. Dilating arteries and veins improves circulation to various body parts. By increasing blood flow to the brain, gingko may help to improve memory in patients with mild memory impairment. Gingko has also been shown to improve blood flow to the peripheral circulation and may help individuals with peripheral vascular disease. Some preliminary reports have shown improved blood flow to the genital area which may help patients with sexual dysfunction due to the side effects of some of the antidepressant drugs such as the serotonin reuptake inhibitors (SRIs). This group of drugs includes paroxetine (Paxil), fluoxetine (Prozac), sertraline (Zoloft), and citolopram (Celexa).

One of gingko's side effects is also clinically significant. It has potent platelet-inhibiting effects and may cause bleeding in patients who are also on other drugs that inhibit clotting. There have been several reports of spontaneous subdural hematomas with chronic use of gingko combined with aspirin. (Jellin JM, Gregory PJ, Butz R, et al. *Natural Medicines Comprehensive Database*. Stockton California: Therapeutic Research Faculty, 2001.) (Borins M. "What to tell your patients about herbs," *Hospital Medicine*, August 1999).

Ginseng. Preliminary studies have shown that taking American ginseng may lower the steep blood sugar rise seen after a meal in patients with type

2 diabetes. The dose was three grams prior to eating, however, one gram will probably do the trick. Is this enough to run out and start gobbling American ginseng? No. First of all, the ginseng used for the study is *not* available as an over-the-counter herbal product. Second, the studies are preliminary and the sample size was a whopping 19 patients. So, hold off on the ginseng until more research has been completed. It's promising, but too early for clinical practice. (Vuksan V. *Archives of Internal Medicine 2000*; 160: 1009)

Girdles. The term girdle is considered archaic these days. Sounds rather old-fashioned and nerdy to wear a girdle so we now wear "molders," "shapers," "smoothers," or "trimmers." Although the name has changed to protect the blubber, the function still remains the same—to hide our bulges, blubber and excess flab.

Glycemic index. The glycemic index (GI) measures how rapidly foods are broken down into glucose or simple sugars. Each food is assigned a glycemic index number, with a high GI number over 70 signifying a rapid rise in blood sugar accompanied by an equally rapid surge in the release of insulin. The faster the insulin is released from the pancreas, the more pounds you pack around your middle. In theory, the more weight you pack around your middle, the higher your risk for type 2 diabetes.

A glycemic index of 100 is pure glucose. Foods with a low glycemic index, less than 55, stimulate a much slower release of insulin and thereby assist in keeping one's lovely 21-inch waistline. Examples of foods with glycemic indexes less than 55 include lentils (28), soybeans (18), apples (38), peaches (42), skim milk (32), heavy, mixed grain bread (30-45), All-Bran cereal (42), low-fat yogurt (33), and a *chocolate bar* (49—yes!). Foods with a glycemic index greater than 70 tend to be low-fiber, highly refined carbohydrates such as white bread (70), Corn Flakes (84), jelly beans (80), Gatorade (78), and watermelon (72). Some foods considered in the "gray zone," between good and bad are bananas (55), ice cream with full fat (61), and a Mars Bar (65). The diet book, *Sugarbusters!* By H. Leighton Steward et al, is based on eliminating foods with a high glycemic index.

Before rushing off to the bookstore to buy various diet books on low glycemic index diets, remember that high glycemic foods are not the only culprit in an ever-increasing waistline, or in the development of type 2 diabetes. Nutrition experts are just beginning to test this theory as well as testing food preparation techniques and how other foods eaten at the same time might influence the glycemic index. Stay tuned.

For more information on the glycemic index, see Appendix B.

Gourmand syndrome. Swiss researchers have reported on a new brain disorder in a small percentage of patients who have suffered strokes, brain tumors, and head trauma. In each case, the damage has produced a persistent behavioral effect—a craving for fine foods. As of today, none of the patients has requested a cure for this condition.

The first patient described with this syndrome was a 48-year-old man who had been hospitalized with a stroke. CT scans pinpointed the area to a small region around the middle cerebral artery in the right frontal hemisphere. He also suffered a temporary weakness on the left side of the body. His main concern, however, was not the temporary inability to ambulate, but with the lousy hospital food. Since this complaint is basically universal in all hospital patients, his fixation on the hospital food was basically ignored. However, when the neuropsychologist asked him to keep a diary of his thoughts, the man exhibited a inordinate preoccupation with food. Before the stroke, he had an overwhelming interest in politics as a political journalist, and very little interest in fine dining. After the stroke, he dumped the political scene and became a columnist for fine dining.

The second patient with gourmand syndrome, a businessman hospitalized for a right-sided, middle cerebral artery stroke, exhibited a new found "lusting" after food. After studying 723 more patients having a similar area involved, the researchers identified 34 more instances of gourmand syndrome. Most of the patients exhibited additional symptoms attributed to right-sided cerebral damage, however these symptoms disappeared for the most part, but the passion for food remained. Most of these patients became preoccupied with shopping, dining rituals, and food preparation. None of the patients became overweight as a result of their fine dining cravings. (*Science News* 1997; 151)

Graham crackers. The Reverend Sylvester Graham, a nineteenth century self-proclaimed nutritionist and naturalist, led a crusade against refined white flour. Graham advocated the use of only whole, coarse grain flour for baking and his name became attached to "graham bread" and "graham crackers," also referred to at the time as "digestive biscuits." Seems like he was a bit before his time as the fiber fanatics have struck again in the twenty-first century.

Grapes. Grapes are perfect for winemaking. They have enough sugar to produce a product that has 10% alcohol and they have enough acid to inhibit the growth of pathogens during the fermentation process. One ton of grapes will make 170 gallons of wine.

Will one glass of nonalcoholic grape juice substitute for one glass of wine's health benefits? Both grapes and red wine contain flavonoids that protect the heart. However, daily wine consumption may be problematic for women because of alcohol's association with an increased risk of breast cancer. The July 2000 issue of the *American Journal of Clinical Nutrition* provides an answer to the question. The researchers suggest that the daily glass of grape juice is just as effective, if not more so, than the glass of wine.

The researchers tested blood levels of antioxidants in volunteers given regular red wine and then the same red wine with the alcohol removed. The antioxidants remained in the blood stream longer with the nonalcoholic wine. They suggest that alcohol may encourage the breakdown and elimination of the antioxidants

Grapefruit. One-half of a pink grapefruit has 1 gram of dietary fiber, 320-780 IU of vitamin A (up to 15.6% of the RDA for a man, and up to 19.5% of the RDA for a woman), and 47 mg of vitamin C (78% of the RDA). White grapefruit isn't quite as nutritious. One-half of a white grapefruit has 1 gram of dietary fiber but only 10 IU of vitamin A, and 39 mg of vitamin C. Pink and red grapefruits are also rich in the carotenoid, lycopene. Lycopene appears to lower the risk of cancer of the prostate gland. Lycopene also appears to lower the risk for heart disease. Another substance in grapefruit, D-limonene, is a member of a family of plant chemicals that also appears to protect against the development of cancer. Remember that foods that are high in vitamin C also help to absorb iron from iron supplements or foods that are rich in iron. The other benefit of grapefruit as well as other foods that are high in vitamin C is that they help to promote wound healing. Vitamin C is necessary for the conversion of proline to hydroxyproline, an essential component of collagen. Collagen is the "glue" that holds skin, bones, and tendons together.

Grapefruit juice or grapefruit, and drugs. Naringin is the alkaloid in the grapefruit that wreaks havoc with the drug metabolizing enzymes in the small intestine. This enzyme system is known as the cytochrome P450 system and the specific enzyme affected is 3A4. Grapefruit *and* grapefruit juice inhibit the ability of this enzyme to initiate the metabolism of drugs in the small intestine. This increases the absorption of the drug in its active form and subsequently increases the risk for drug side effects. The number of drugs interacting with grapefruit juice is astronomical. The list in Appendix C is not inclusive, but gives you an idea of the wide spectrum of drug classes and specific drugs affected by grapefruit juice. As a general rule, concomitant administration of grapefruit juice with these drugs should be avoided. See Appendix C.

Grapefruit juice and kidney stones. Women can significantly reduce their risk for kidney stones by drinking wine and tea. Using data from the Nurses' Health Study, researchers from Brigham and Women's Hospital and Harvard School of Public Health and Medical School showed consumption of tea, coffee (with and without caffeine), and wine can reduce the risk of kidney stones.

After controlling for a zillion variables, the researchers found one cup of coffee or tea daily or one glass of wine decreased the risk of kidney stones by 8% (tea and coffee) and by 59% (wine). Clearly the drink of the hour here is wine, wine, fruit of the vine.

On the other hand, consuming grapefruit juice had just the opposite effect. One 8-ounce glass of grapefruit juice increased the risk of kidney stones by 44%. Clearly the drink not to choose is grapefruit juice. (*Annals of Internal Medicine;* April 1, 1998.)

GRILLING

Grilling temperatures to kill the bugs. According to the FDA, the minimum safe temperature for various types of foods, however they are cooked, is as follows (in degrees Fahrenheit):

Ground beef, veal, lamb, and pork—160°

Beef, veal, lamb (steaks, chops, and roasts)—145°

Pork (roast and chops)—160°

Ham, uncooked—160°

Ham, precooked—140°

Ground chicken and turkey—165°

Whole chicken and turkey—180°

Poultry breasts—170°

Poultry thighs and wings—180°

Poultry stuffing (cooked alone or in the bird)—165°
Egg dishes and casseroles—160°
Leftovers—165°

NOTE: Reheated soups and gravies should be brought to a rolling boil; all other leftovers should be hot and steaming.

Remember that the only way you can safely know if the meat is cooked is to use a thermometer. Just eyeballing the meat doesn't do the trick. For measuring the temperature after it comes out of the oven or off the grill, a digital thermometer is best, since it needs to be inserted only half an inch and it records the temperature in just 10 seconds. For measuring the foods while they are still in the oven, either a liquid-filled or bimetal oven-safe thermometer (the old stand-by) is useful.

One last note: If you are nervous about under-cooking fish, here's a helpful hint from the May, 2000 *Nutrition Action Newsletter*. Measure the the thickness of any fillet at its thickest point. Cook it 10 minutes per inch. It doesn't matter if you are baking, broiling, grilling, steaming or poaching the fish.

Guaiac test for occult blood in the stool. Certain foods can interact with the guaiac test for hidden (occult) blood in feces. The active ingredient in the guaiac slide test is alphaguaiaconic acid, a chemical that turns blue in the presence of blood. Foods containing peroxidase, a natural chemical that also turns alphaguaiaconic acid blue, may produce a false positive test. In other words, the individual will have a positive test without hidden blood in the stool. Foods that cause a false positive test include: Artichokes, broccoli, carrots, cauliflower, cucumbers, lamb, mushrooms, oranges or other citrus fruits and vitamin supplements that contain more than 250 mg of vitamin C, radishes, and turnips. These foods should be eliminated from the diet for three days prior to testing for blood in the stool.

Gum chewing and GERD (Gastroesophageal reflux disease) prevention. Chew gum to stimulate saliva—it helps to neutralize the gastric acid that is refluxing from the stomach into the lower esophagus. Drink fluids between meals, not with meals. Combining fluids with foods increases the likelihood of reflux.

Gum chewing and headaches. Yet another trigger for migraines. The journal *Headache*, has listed yet another trigger for migraine headaches. After chewing sugarless gum, patients experienced throbbing headaches. The culprit was determined to be aspartame—the sweetener used in sugarless gum.

Gum chewing and weight loss. People who continuously chew sugarless gum burn 11 calories more per hour than people who sit still and do nothing. This translates into a weight loss of about 10 pounds over a year, if calorie intake stays the same. (*New England Journal of Medicine*, December 30, 1999.)

GUSTATORY RHINITIS

Gustatory rhinitis—the "Salsa Sniffles." Gustatory rhinitis, also known as the "Salsa Sniffles," occurs when one snarfs down meals containing chili peppers, horseradish sauce, onions and other spicy hot foods. These sniffles and drips are due to over-stimulated parasympathetic (cholinergic) nerves that supply the glands in the nasal passages. Fluid production is turned on and the drip begins.

Garlic Toast
Makes 4 servings

ina's
breakfast · lunch · dinner

        2 tsp. olive oil
       12 slices (1/2 inch thick) diagonally cut French baguette
        1 garlic clove, halved

If you have a cast iron grill pan, or just a heavy fry pan, heat over medium-high heat.

With a pastry brush or your hand, cover the cut sides of the bread evenly with the olive oil.

Place the bread in the pan and cook for about a minute on each side or until lightly browned.

Rub the garlic clove on one side of the bread.

Nutritional info: Serving is 3 pieces of bread: Calories 79; Total fat 2.9gr.; Protein 2.2gr.; Carbohydrates 12.7 gr.; Fiber 1 gr.; Sodium 133 gr.

H

is for...

Hamburger Hell

Hamburger Hell.. Recent studies have revealed that approximately 23-28% of the cattle in the U.S. are colonized with the deadly mutant form of *E. Coli* known as *E. Coli O157:H7*. Less than five years ago only 1% of our cows were infected. Some important notes about this deadly pathogen include the following:

- *E. Coli O157:H7* is infectious at low doses. Comparing the infectivity dose with cholera emphasizes the difference. Whereas cholera requires the presence of 10,000,000 to 100,000,000 organisms before clinical illness occurs, *E. Coli* can produce clinical symptoms with as few as 10-100 organisms.
- *E. Coli O157:H7* is referred to as acid-tolerant, therefore the normally protective high acid pH of the stomach will not destroy this bacteria as it passes through this first line of defense.
- *E. Coli O157:H7* is unaffected by freezing, however, it cannot survive for long at temperatures warmer than 120° F (49° C).
- Most slab meat is safe because the *E. ColiO157:H7* organisms are only found on the exterior of the meat and are easily killed during the cooking process.
- Hamburger meat is the real culprit due to the method by which it is processed. Ground meat, with *ground* being the operative word, is produced from the "trimmings" or remnants of higher-grade cuts of meat. These remnants are mixed together in a big vat with the scraps of other animals from different sources and are subsequently ground together. This grinding process is a highly efficient way of distributing *E. ColiO157: H7* throughout the ground meat. As a result, each hamburger patty may be chock-full of the bacteria. If the burger patty is not thoroughly cooked at temps above 120° F, the organisms at the center of the patty can remain viable and cause significant disease.

- Forming contaminated ground beef into hamburger patties can leave a residue of about 10 million *E. Coli O157:H7* on your hands. Another reason to wash your hands, eh? In fact, this form of *E. Coli* can survive on a stainless steel countertop for up to 60 days. So, clean those countertops and cutting boards with soap and water and don't prepare other foods in the same area that you form those hamburger patties.
- Flash back to the Jack-in-the-Box outbreak in Seattle-Tacoma, Washington in 1993. Investigators concluded that the burgers causing the most illness had been cooked at the edges of the grill and had not reached the required temperature to kill the bacteria.
- Estimates of the percentage of burgers sold that now contain detectable levels of *E. Coli* range between 0.1-1% to 4-10%.
- Hamburger meat is the major culprit in the majority of outbreaks, however, alfalfa sprouts, lettuce, and unpasteurized apple ciders have all been responsible for outbreaks.
- Frank bloody diarrhea is the hallmark of *E. Coli O157:H7* infection. Keep it in mind whenever a patient reports bloody diarrhea. At some centers a CBC and differential are routinely recommended to look for evidence of hemolysis. Be alert for danger signs such as a fall in the patient's platelet count or a decrease in urinary output.

HISTORICAL HIGHLIGHT

Even though the esteemed *Oxford English Dictionary* traces the first reference to the hamburger to 1889, the residents of Seymour, Wisconsin beg to differ. As the story goes, 15-year-old Charlie Nagreen arrived at the Seymour-Outagamie County fair in 1885 in an ox-drawn wagon with plans to open a food stand that sold fried meatballs. Well, fried meatballs weren't "in" that year and no one seemed to be interested. Actually the problem was in the presentation—it's hard to stroll around the fairgrounds eating meatballs. So, Charlie decided to flatten the meatballs and plopped the flattened meat in between two pieces of bread and voilá! Hamburger. Charlie became a legend in his own right. He returned to the Seymour-Outagamie County Fair every year after that, for 65 years and made the rounds at all of the other county fairs in Wisconsin. Seymour, Wisconsin's claim to fame is the 5,520-pound grilled hamburger patty made in 1989 to celebrate the centennial (based on the *Oxford English Dictionary's* definition which of course, is still in dispute). The residents of Seymour are currently raising the big bucks, to the tune of $15 million, to build a four-story, hamburger-shaped shrine. **Hamburger Hall of Fame, 126 N. Main Street, Seymour, Wisconsin 54165. 414-833-9522**

- The use of antibiotics is discouraged. Antibiotics kill the bacteria in the bowel and cause the release of toxins. The use of antibiotics has been associated with an increase in the incidence of hemolytic uremic syndrome and acute kidney (renal) failure in kids.

Qadri SM, Kayalis S. "*Enterohemorrhagic E. Coli.*" Postgraduate Medicine 1998; 103(2):179-87. Buchanan RL, et al. "The rising tide of foodborne and waterborne infections." Patient Care 1997; May 15:31-72.

Hamburger "heaven." Hamburgers and cheeseburgers account for 76% of all the beef sold in restaurants. Steak accounts for just 5%. As a staple of the general diet, ground beef accounts for approximately 45% of the beef we eat. The average American consumed 27 pounds of ground beef in 1997. That is the equivalent to a Quarter Pounder from Mickey D's every three days. Even though we consider hamburgers our meat of choice here in the U.S., it's not the best choice. It contributes more than 60% of the saturated fat we get from beef. It has also most likely contributed to quite a few extra pounds around our middle as well as to quite a few clogged arteries along the way.

"If you had to pick a single food that inflicts the most damage on the American diet, ground beef would be a prime contender. Whether it's tacos, meatloaf, lasagna, or the ubiquitous hamburger, Americans stuff themselves with ground beef without a second thought about its consequences."
—Nutrition Action Newsletter, September 1999.

Hamburgers on the grill. Flip those burgers every 60 seconds for safety's sake. While all cooking methods reduce the levels of *E. Coli O157:H7* in raw ground beef, turning the patties every minute did it faster. As an extra-added bonus, your burgers will cook faster. The frequent-flipping method cooked the burgers in 8 minutes compared to a 16-minute cooking time when the burgers were turned over just once after 5 minutes of cooking.

Hamburgers, holes and White Castles—the scoop on "Sliders." At last, the answer to your question as to why White Castle hamburgers have five holes per patty. The holes were introduced in 1946 (twenty-five years after the first White Castle was up and running in 1921 in Wichita, Kansas), for a very important reason. The holes allow the steam and grease from the grill to escape *up* the holes to the upper bun, which cooks atop each patty. This release of steam and grease eliminates the need to flip over the meat in order to cook it evenly. How simple is that?

The Halimeter. This new device measures the level of bacteria in the mouth. Used exclusively in the "fresh breath" clinics in California, the halimeter is the first step in determining the cause and severity of halitosis. Once the level of bacteria has been measured, the tongue scrapers, tooth irrigators, and other bacteria-removing devices are employed to rid the oral cavity of the bugs that contribute to *bad breath*.

Halitosis. Bad breath usually develops during sleep when the salivary glands that produce 500-1,000 milliliters of saliva during waking hours slow production to just under 10 milliliters at night. The mouth becomes a stagnant reservoir of 1,600 billion bacterial flora that feast on dead buccal cells and remaining filet mignon from the evening meal. The bacteria break down the cells and food particles into sulfur compounds, imparting that early morning "boiled egg" breath. The cure—brush your teeth and scrape the tongue before bedtime.

Hormonal fluctuations also play a role in the development of halitosis. Women have more of a problem during ovulation. The increase in estrogen causes the blood vessels in the gum surrounding each tooth to contract, forming a crevice that allows fluid to pool, attracting bacteria.

To increase salivary flow, and decrease halitosis, eat an orange or grapefruit between meals. It gives your mouth's natural cleansing system a boost.

If halitosis persists after scraping the back of the tongue with a teaspoon, try a nonprescription tablet of bismuth subgallate from the American Foundation for Preventive Medicine, P.O. Box 1144, Indianapolis, IN 46202.

Ham. The term "ham" is used loosely, however, it technically refers to the hind leg of a pig, from the shank to the hip. You can define hams further by the type of pig, to the curing method, to the smoking time, to the region in which the ham is made. For example, *Country ham* is the result of a long curing process in which the ham is smoked over fragrant hardwoods and aged for up to one year. No water is added during the process, resulting in a highly flavored, salty ham. You can have a delicious slice of this ham at any roadside diner in the southern part of the U.S. If you drive through Smithfield County, Virginia, you may recognize the home of the premier cured and processed *Smithfield* country ham. *Prosciutto* is an Italian ham that is salted and air-dried but not smoked. It is usually served in paper-thin slices and wrapped around a delicious piece of cantaloupe. *Canned ham* is made from either a whole piece of meat or it is "formed" from smaller pieces of meat. It is brine-cured, pressed, and molded, often with the addition of gelatin to help retain the natural juices. *Cottage ham* or *smoked Boston shoulder* comes from the neck and shoulder of the pig, not the leg. It has also been called the *daisy ham*. *Fresh ham* is another term that refers to a cut from the shoulder of the pig. It is uncooked and has a delicate pork flavor that lacks the smokiness or saltiness of cured hams. And how could I forget to mention the number one canned luncheon meat sold around the world, SPAM.

What exactly is SPAM? The term SPAM comes from the combination of two words, SPiced hAM. It consists of a loaf of molded ground pork shoulder with some added ground ham, salt, H_2O, sugar, and sodium nitrite. The amount of sodium in one 2-oz. serving of SPAM is enough to make any blood pressure skyrocket. This 2-oz. serving contains 750 mg of sodium, 170 calories, with 140 of those calories from saturated fat.. SPAM is death in a can. Thank goodness for SPAM LITE. It's 25% *less* sodium, and 140 calories, 90% of which are saturated fats. Remarkably, SPAM does not make the top 10 food list at Weight Watcher's.

The George A. Hormel Company of Austin, Minnesota, manufactures SPAM. *Who Eats SPAM?* There must be a few million closet SPAM eaters in this world because eighty-five million pounds of canned SPAM are sold per year which equates to 75% of the canned luncheon meat market in the U.S. and overseas. How many of you are drooling over the possibility of a SPAM and cheese sandwich as we speak?

Well, the pork packers of the world might be the only ones. In their journal, *Squeal,* an article called the introduction of SPAM to the world as "historic" as the first rifle shot at the Battle of Lexington. In the "What's on the Menu" section of the journal, the following recipes were found: Polynesian Baked SPAM, Sweet and Sour SPAM, SPAM enchilada breakfast casserole, and Spaghetti Carbonara with SPAM, cool SPAM, cucumber and avocado sandwiches. And if you don't have *Squeal* on your coffee table you can go to your local bookstore and purchase the definitive cookbook on every SPAM recipe known to man. Dorothy Horn has published a SPAM cookbook with over 500 recipes.

The island of Guam wins the prize for the most SPAM consumed in the world per year and per capita. Guam has 135,000 citizens, but consumes 1.5 million cans of SPAM per year.

HAND WASHING

Hand washing. "With the possible exception of immunization," says Ralph Cordell, an epidemiologist at the Centers for Disease Control and

Prevention in Atlanta, "hand-washing is the most effective disease-preventing measure anyone can practice."

Studies have shown that a single hand can carry around 200 million organisms, including bacteria, viruses, and a few fungi thrown in for good measure. It takes a *full* five minutes of hand washing to cleanse 99% of the most dangerous bacteria from the fingernails, thumbs, palm creases, and backs of the hands. Surgeons have the time to do this, the rest of us do not. So, if you want to wash off 95% of the bugs lurking in the nooks and crannies of your hands, wash to the tune of "Twinkle, Twinkle, Little Star."

A recent study observing emergency room physicians and nurses found that they washed their hands less than a third of the time after touching patients. And when they did take the time to use soap and water, the average wash-and-rinse was a mere 9.5 seconds. The good news: *E.Coli* and other intestinal bugs are the first to go with soap and water—they exit the hands after about five seconds of the wash. Plain soap and water also "uncoat" the flu virus, rendering it incapable of infecting cells of the respiratory tract.

Another interesting tidbit—the hand you use the most, the dominant hand, is often under-washed. If you're right-handed, your left hand is usually cleaner.

So, if you're in a hurry (who isn't?), clean your hands with an alcohol gel fortified with a skin-protecting emollient like glycerin, or wipe your hands with an alcohol-laden towelette. Research has shown that alcohol hand rinses are actually much better at getting rid of bacteria than soap. (Williams G. "The Biology of Hand-Washing".) *Discover Magazine.* December 1999; 36-38)

Finally, when asked directly, 98% of women claim they wash their hands after using the restroom. When observed directly, only 74% actually do. Tsk...Tsk..

Hepatitis A. Hepatitis caused by the Hepatitis A virus (HAV) is contracted through contaminated food or water. Young adults and children in institutional settings and travelers in countries with minimal sanitation are at greatest risk for infection; small epidemics have been seen among persons eating at restaurants that served contaminated shellfish. The course of the illness is usually mild, with the acute stage resolving in about 2 weeks and complete recovery within 8 weeks. When traveling to countries with poor sanitation consider the Hepatitis A vaccine to develop immunity or the immunoglobulin to HAV for acute protection. Also use good clinical judgment about the foods you choose and the water you drink, depending on the country.

Hepatitis C Virus (HCV). Is there a special diet for patients with chronic hepatitis C? If a person has cirrhosis as a complication of Hepatitis C, it is recommended that they steer clear of raw seafood, iron, and limit or avoid vitamin A supplements. In addition, certain herbal products have been found to be toxic to the liver and should be avoided at all costs in patients with chronic liver disease. These herbal supplements include chaparral, comfrey, germander, jin bu huan, mistletoe, nutmeg, ragwort, sassafras, senna, and tansy.

If a person with HCV takes a multivitamin, be sure that it is iron-free. The best bet for a patient with Hepatitis C is to consume a diet high in fresh vegetables and fruits, making sure that appropriate safety precautions are taken with washing the vegetables and fruits. It is controversial as to whether or not animal protein should be eliminated from the diet. Most patients can eliminate animal proteins from their diet, however, patients with HCV that are coinfected with HIV cannot. Animal proteins are necessary to keep the immune system healthy in order to fight the HIV infection. (*National AIDS Treatment Advocacy Project Handbook,* NATAP, 580 Broadway, Suite 1010, New York, NY, 10012. www.natap.org)

Herbal products. Before taking any herbal product, check with your health care professional or a certified herbalist near you. Call 1-800-423-8800 for an herbalist in your neck of the woods. See Appendix B.

High Density Lipoproteins (HDLs). To date, most studies have focused on lowering total cholesterol and low-density lipoprotein cholesterol levels to reduce the risk of coronary artery disease and atherosclerosis. The significance of HDL (High Density Lipoprotein) has received less attention. Studies that have focused specifically on HDL have found that low HDL levels are an independent risk factor for coronary artery disease, especially in a high-fat consuming culture such as ours in the U.S. Now, as more and more compelling data are reported, it is necessary to focus on ways to increase HDL levels. Here are some pearls you should know about HDL.

- The risk of coronary artery disease in women is more closely related to the low HDL than to elevated LDL levels.
- The risk of coronary artery disease increases by 2-3% for every 1 mg/dL decrease in HDL.

- HDL protects against atherogenesis (developing fat plaques in the arteries) through at least two mechanisms. First, HDL mediates the removal of excess cholesterol from peripheral tissues, such as blood vessels, and moves it back to the liver through a process known as reverse cholesterol transport. Cholesterol is then excreted from the body through the GI tract in bile. Therefore, higher HDL levels allow for more excretion of excess cholesterol. Second, HDL inhibits the oxidation of LDL. Oxidation of LDL is the first step in the process of fat plaque formation. HDL may also inhibit the migration of the white blood cells known as the monocytes into the inner layer of the artery. Monocytes first engulf LDL and then proceed to "oxidize" it.
- Secondary causes of low HDL include genetic disorders, obesity, smoking cigarettes, drugs, and dietary influences. The major dietary influence that decreases HDL are the trans fatty acids. Trans fatty acids, commonly used in baked goods like cakes, pies, and cookies.
- Moderate exercise (walking a minimum of seven miles per week) does *not* raise HDL levels significantly. However, intense exercise (*running* a minimum of seven miles per week) does increase HDL.
- The positive effects of moderate alcohol intake on heart disease are numerous. Moderate alcohol intake boosts HDL. One study showed that men who abstained from alcohol had an average HDL of 38 mg/dL while those who drank more than 14 drinks per week (2 per day) had an average HDL of 46.2 mg/dL. Alcohol also lowers fibrinogen levels and inhibits platelet aggregation, both of which contribute to the inhibition of clotting and reduce the risk of heart attacks.
- HDL levels are inversely related to Body Mass Index (BMI). Does weight loss increase HDL? Apparently weight loss through diet alone, does *not*. However, the literature supports the position that weight loss through exercise raises HDL. This finding is specifically *for men only*. Women have been found to have decreases in HDL when losing weight by diet alone. The decreases in HDL were less significant among women who also exercised to lose weight.
- Soy products lower LDL levels but their effect on HDL is less clear. A recent study found that 25 to 50 grams of soy protein per day only increased HDL levels by 2.4%.
- Replacing saturated fat calories with carbohydrates has a negative effect on HDL levels. However, replacing saturated fats with monosaturated fats (olive oil) maintains HDL levels and also lowers the incidence of heart disease. Patients with isolated low HDL levels should be cautioned against drastically cutting total dietary fat and should instead be encouraged to replace saturated fat with monosaturated fats such as olive oil and canola oil.
- Lifestyle changes (more exercise, smoking cessation, moderate alcohol consumption) increase HDL by about 10-15%.

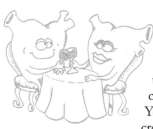

Holiday heart. Heart attacks occur in a seasonal pattern. A research team from UCLA examined the month-by-month death rate from myocardial infarctions over a 12-year period. They found that it stayed relatively stable through November and then increased dramatically after Thanksgiving and peaked around New Year's Day. The incidence of heart attacks increased by 33% in December and January.

One would perhaps assume that the winter trigger for heart attacks would be cold weather and subsequent coronary vasoconstriction resulting in an increased workload on the heart. However, upon closer scrutiny of the data, the authors of the study realized that even in warm areas such as Southern California where the temperatures rarely dip below 50° F, even on the coldest day of the year, there was still an increase in the number of heart attacks.

The second theory blames the good old American way of overindulging during the holiday season—lots of booze, fatty foods, and salt to make the season bright. A heavy meal quadruples the risk for a heart attack. It temporarily raises blood pressure, which may rupture a cholesterol-laden plaque already present. A heavy meal also increases insulin, which can make coronary arteries less relaxed. The increased stress of the holiday season increases cortisol levels which in turn increase blood glucose and increase the stickiness of platelets, making platelets more likely to clot. (*Circulation* 2000; 1(02) (Supplement):612.)

NOTE: Just in case you were wondering, the lowest-risk month for heart attacks is June with September second and July and August coming in third and fourth.

H
115

Homocysteine: Yet another important risk factor for heart disease.

What the heck is homocysteine? Homocysteine is an amino acid that is normally converted to one of two other amino acids, methionine or cysteine. This normal metabolic process depends on adequate amounts of 22 vitamins belonging to the B-family. The most important of the family are B6, B12, and folic acid. Deficiencies of any of the three nutrients may lead to excess homocysteine, as defined by a level of greater than 11 micromoles per liter, which in turn promotes the development of atherosclerosis.

How does homocysteine protect you from heart disease? Excess homocysteine has been shown to inhibit an important enzyme in the vascular smooth muscle. This enzyme, glutathione peroxide, is necessary to prevent vascular smooth muscle proliferation, which has been shown to contribute to the development of atherosclerotic plaque formation. In addition, elevated levels of homocysteine may also impair the release of a potent vasodilator, nitric oxide. This contributes to the process by elevating intra-arterial pressure, another important risk factor for atherosclerotic plaque formation. And a third consequence of elevated homocysteine levels is the activation of protein C, which subsequently triggers the clotting cascade.

Are elevated homocysteine levels a rare finding or a finding that primary care practitioners should be concerned about? In the past five years, studies of more than 17,000 patients have indicated that cardiovascular risk increases directly with any increase in homocysteine level, much as it does with any increase in total serum cholesterol level. One study, the Physician's Health Study (a prospective study of almost 15,000 physicians), revealed the relative risk of myocardial infarction or death from coronary heart disease was 3.4 for those physicians whose homocysteine levels were in the highest five%. The risk of heart disease doubles for each 5-point increase in homocysteine levels. Elevated homocysteine levels have also been associated with peripheral vascular disease and carotid atherosclerosis.

Should all patients be tested for homocysteine levels? No, this is not currently recommended, however, it may be appropriate to obtain the homocysteine level in patients with premature heart disease who lack traditional risk factors such as smoking, hypertension, elevated LDL-cholesterol, low HDL-cholesterol, obesity, and a sedentary lifestyle. A recommendation for testing may be forthcoming, however, especially in light of a recent study published in the *Archives of Internal Medicine* . This study estimated that 32% of the women over age 50 have elevated homocysteine levels that put them at increased risk for heart disease. The study analyzed the costs and benefits of screening men and women for elevated homocysteine as well as treating elevations of the amino acid with inexpensive vitamins. They found that treatment with B-vitamins, B6, folic acid, and B12, in particular could save thousands of dollars in health care costs due to the reduction in heart disease complications.

Can high homocysteine levels be prevented or treated, once established? Yes, indeed. The good news is that supplementation with just 1 mg of folic acid per day can reduce homocysteine levels by as much as 42%. In addition, adding just 1 mg of B12 to the regimen daily would alleviate concern that the administration of folate might mask B12 deficiency. And, last but not least, 2 mg per day of vitamin B6 has also been shown to reduce elevated levels of homocysteine. For more information see Appendix B.

Homocysteine and Alzheimer's disease. Not only are high homocysteine levels linked with an increased risk of coronary artery disease, recent studies have also implicated high levels in association with Alzheimer's disease. Researchers in England followed 164 patients diagnosed with Alzeimer's disease. Compared with age- and sex-matched controls, those with

Alzheimer's had significantly lower levels of nutrients that reduce homocysteine—folic acid and B12. This study doesn't actually prove that high homocysteine contributes to an increased Alzheimer's risk, or that B12 can help prevent the disease. However, it does contribute to a growing body of evidence that one component of Alzheimer's disease is a type of vascular disease and shares risk factors with other vascular conditions.

"The pessimist is someone who can look at the land of milk and honey and see only calories and cholesterol. —Quote magazine

Honey is a "no-no" for infants. Eating honey in both natural and processed forms, can lead to serious disease and even death in infants. Because of the environment in which it's produced, unprocessed honey often contains spores of *Clostridium botulinum,* the bacterium that causes botulism. The same can be true for processed honey. In most humans, the spores cause no problems; immune cells in the GI tracts of older children and adults release binding proteins that neutralize the toxin. The GI tracts of children under one year of age are too immature to produce the proteins needed to neutralize and destroy the toxin. Once the toxin enters the bloodstream after being absorbed through the GI tract, it binds to receptors on skeletal muscle and results in paralysis. Within hours of ingesting the contaminated honey, infants become lethargic, flaccid and can develop respiratory arrest. If the diagnosis is made early, the prognosis for a full recovery is excellent.

Honey is a "yes-yes" for hangover headaches. Here's a tip for preventing and/or managing a hangover headache. Eat some honey. Spread it on a cracker or over some toast, before or after the alcohol, and you may prevent the inevitable headache from being "over-served." Honey supplies fructose, which helps the body metabolize alcohol and reduce hangover symptoms. If you do wind up with a headache, even after this prudent advice, drink fluids containing minerals and salts to alleviate the dehydration from the alcohol. For example, a cup of bouillon replaces fluids and does not cause nausea. And the vasoconstrictor effects of a quick hit of java (coffee), help to shorten the duration of the headache. (National Headache Foundation, Chicago, IL)

Honeymoon. One of the customs of the day, 4,000 years ago in far away Babylon, was for the father of the bride to supply the new son-in-law with all the mead he could drink for the first month of marriage. Since mead is a honey beer and because the calendar was based on the cycle of the moon, this period was referred to as the "Honey Month" or what is commonly known today as the "Honeymoon."

Hospital food. Just the mere mention of hospital food sends chills up and down the spine…and now, a study has given us another reason for those chills, besides the obvious. A national survey of 57 university hospitals found that the menus at only 7% met all the federal dietary guidelines. Of menus for patients with no dietary restrictions, 40% served too much fat, and more than half poured on the salt. So much for practicing what we preach.

Hot dogs. What would a summer be without hot dogs? What would a baseball game be without hot dogs? The connection between baseball and

HISTORICAL HIGHLIGHT

The National Hot Dog and Sausage Council says that European immigrants first brought hot dogs to the United States from Germany and Austria in the 1800s. The frankfurter was nicknamed dachshund dog because of its resemblance to the little canine. Legend has it that the term "hot dog" was coined at the Polo Grounds during a baseball game around 1906. Concessionaire Harry M. Stevens couldn't sell ice cream and soda on a cold day in April, so he had his vendors load up on sausages and hollar, "Get your red hot dachshund dogs!" It just so happened that a cartoonist for the *New York Journal* was at the park looking for an idea and penned an illustration of a real dachshund in a bun with the caption, "Get your hot dogs!" As the story goes, the cartoonist, Tad Dorgan, couldn't spell dachshund, so he shortened the caption to just "hot dogs." Unfortunately, no one can find the cartoon by Tad Dorgan, so the story has been disputed. Now the ballpark and hot dog historians are back at the drawing board as to the origins of the hot dog.

hot dogs has a 100-year history. The origin of the connection is unknown, but it is a well-established fact that hot dog carts have ruled ballparks for more than a century. Baseball fans will eat nearly 27 million hot dogs in major league parks during the summer of 2001, according to the National Hot Dog and Sausage Council. In fact, string all those "dawgs" together and you can link Yankee Stadium with the Dodger's Stadium in Los Angeles.

The San Francisco Giants offered a tofu hot dog for two years but didn't get many takers. The National Hot Dog and Sausage council has its own name for the tofu frank—The Weakest Link.

"A hot dog at the ballpark is better than steak at the Ritz."
— Humphrey Bogart

HISTORICAL HIGHLIGHT

Where did the term originate, *to eat humble pie?* This saying dates back to the eighteenth century. The men of the house were given the best meat of any meal (filet, T-bone, sirloin) and of course, the women and children ate the umbles or leftovers, the tongue and the entrails (the intestines). The leftovers were baked in an *umble pie*, hence the name.

HYPERTENSION

Hypertension and women. Women who drink more than 30 grams of alcohol per day (about 2 ½ drinks) have a 32% increase in the risk of developing hypertension.

The more fruits and vegetables consumed by women, the lower the blood pressure. One daily serving of tofu reduces the systolic blood pressure by 2.6 mmHg and the diastolic by 0.7 mmHg. Add a little spinach to the tofu and reduce the systolic blood pressure by an additional 1.7 mmHg and the diastolic by an additional .8 mmHg. Brown rice tops the list— one daily serving reduces the systolic BP by 3 mmHg and the diastolic by 1 mmHg. The bottom line: Tofu, spinach, and brown rice appear to be your best bet for not only blood pressure reduction but also for the most unappetizing meal of the day.

Magnesium-containing foods (legumes, nuts, grains, dark-green leafy vegetables, cocoa, dried fruits, shellfish) and fiber (barley, brown rice, apples, prunes, corn, potatoes with skins, yams, legumes and nuts) will also help lower blood pressure. Potassium and calcium have also been shown to reduce blood pressure. Potassium-containing foods include potatoes, prunes, oranges, cantaloupes, bananas and of course, the calcium-containing foods are milk and milk products, yogurt, cheeses, broccoli and sardines. (*Harvard Health Letter* Vol. 7(1): September 1996)

Hypoglycemia. Hypoglycemia is the most common endocrine emergency seen by primary care practitioners. It frequently occurs in patients receiving insulin treatment with tight control of their diabetes and in older patients receiving a sulfonylurea drug, such as glyburide or glipizide. Another common group are people who have nonspecific symptoms including fatigue, concentration difficulties, anxiety and dizziness. Most of the time these patients are self-diagnosed and will need a workup by the primary care practitioner or endocrinologist to determine the cause of the hypoglycemia.

Clinical hypoglycemia is defined using the following criteria:
- Central nervous system symptoms including confusion, aberrant behavior, seizures, and coma.
- A simultaneous blood glucose level equal to or less than 40 mg/dL.
- Relief of these symptoms by the administration of glucose.

An abrupt decrease in blood sugar results in an adrenergic or adrenalin response. The blood glucose does not necessarily have to fall below 40 mg/dL for the patient to experience symptom. The patient may complain of headache, slurred speech, confusion, tremors, tachycardia, and the inability to concentrate. The metabolic effect of adrenalin includes glycogenolysis, or the breakdown of stored sugar (glycogen) in the liver. Once the glycogen is metabolized it turns into pure glucose, giving the blood sugar a metabolic boost.

The longer the patient has diabetes, the less obvious are the signs and symptoms of hypoglycemia. Patients who have had diabetes for more than 10 years may not manifest with the classic signs listed above. Instead, numbness and /or tingling (around the mouth especially), yawning and or a feeling of "heaviness" in the legs may become primary symptoms.

Ten to fifteen grams of a fast acting carbohydrate will increase the blood sugar most rapidly. The recommended source for the fast-acting carbohydrate is a cup of skim milk. If skim milk isn't handy, four ounces of fruit juice will do, as will 6-7 pieces of hard candy or 4 ounces of regular cola.

One mistake that is commonly made is to add 5 packs of sugar to an 8-ounce glass of orange juice. This definitely is "overkill" as far as a sugar dose is concerned. Another common mistake is to use ice cream or a chocolate bar to treat the hypoglycemia. The large fat content of these foods slows the absorption of the sugar so that the blood glucose level does not rise as rapidly, putting the patient in danger of more prolonged hypoglycemia.

Horseradish Relish
Makes 4 cups

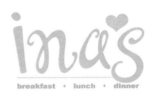

breakfast · lunch · dinner

6	beets, large – trimmed
1	horseradish root, medium
6	cups water
1/4	cup sugar
1/4	cup white vinegar
3/4	tsp. kosher salt

Put the beets and water in a pan and bring to a boil over medium-high heat. Reduce to a simmer and cook about 20 minutes until the beets are tender. Drain and cool.

Peel the beets and coarsely grate them into a large bowl. Grate the horseradish root into the beets.

Dissolve the sugar in the vinegar and stir into beet mixture. Add the salt and taste. Adjust seasonings.

Nutritional Info: Serving size 1 Tablespoon: Calories 5; Total fat 0 gr.; Protein 0.1 gr.; Carbohydrates 1.2 gr.; Fiber 0.1 gr.; Sodium 23 mg.

is for...
Ice Cream, You Scream

Ice cream headache. An ice cream headache is triggered when a cold substance hits the hard palate. Ice cream drastically cools the mouth, triggering vasodilation to increase blood flow and warm up the area. As the blood moves in to warm up the mouth, nerve endings are irritated. The pain peaks in approximately 25-60 seconds, and the skin temperature in the forehead falls almost two degrees Fahrenheit. What is the treatment? Eat your ice cream slowly.

HISTORICAL HIGHLIGHT

Ice cream sodas were quite popular in the late 1800s. Ice cream sodas were made with a mixture of sweet cream, syrup, and carbonated water. In October 1874 a man named Robert Green was selling soda fountain drinks when he ran out of sweet cream. A quick thinker, he decided to use ice cream instead, hoping that no one would notice the substitution. It seems as if everyone noticed. His profits jumped from $6.00 per day selling the traditional ice cream soda to $600.00 per day for the ice cream soda with ice cream added.

The ice cream drink became so popular that religious leaders declared it sinful. By the 1890s some cities and towns passed laws prohibiting the sale of sodas on Sunday. For this reason the ice cream Sundae was invented. (It was spelled with an "ae" so as not to offend the pillars of the Church.)

FACT: The largest ice cream sundae on record weighed 24.5 tons. The sundae was made by Palm Dairies Ltd, under the supervision of Mike Rogiani in Edmonton, Alberta, Canada, on July 24, 1988. (*Guiness World Records,* 2001)

In Sutherland, Iowa, citizens may not carry ice-cream cones in their pockets.

·

In Halstead, KS, residents must refrain from eating ice cream with a fork in public.

INSECT FRAGMENTS

Insect fragments. A new assay is being tested to determine the number of insect fragments in grain products. The current process is to do a gross inspection by spreading out grain kernels and eyeballing them for whole insects or insect fragments—the wing, torso, leg, etc. To pick out the smaller segments, they cook up this elaborate concoction, shake it up, filter off what floats to the top, dry the extract, and look at it under the microscope. Just so you realize the complexity of the job, "It takes six months of training to become an insect fragment counter," says Dr. Barrie Kitto, Chief Insect Fragment Counter.

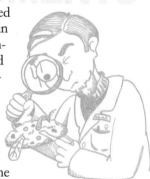

Current federal standards allow 75 insect fragments per 50 grams of grain, but here's the clincher, fragment size. Whether it's three-fourths of a large maggot or just a measly fruit fly's wing tip, is immaterial.

The new assay measures myosin, a muscle protein present in insects at all life stages. When an extraction fluid is added to grain or foods containing the myosin, the mix turns green. The deeper the hue, the greater the amount of myosin found in the grain. Using a color meter, one can quantitate each reading.

INSULIN

Insulin resistance and Syndrome X. What is insulin resistance? The pancreas secretes plenty of insulin but the tissues are resistant to the effects of that insulin. The pancreas tries to compensate by releasing more insulin and a vicious cycle ensues. The excess insulin manages to keep the blood glucose in check however, the glucose level is usually in the upper range of normal. As insulin levels increase so do triglycerides, blood pressure, and levels of small, dense LDL-cholesterol. As all of those parameters rise, the HDL levels plummet.

Syndrome X is also referred to as The Metabolic Syndrome. It occurs in individuals who are insulin resistant. Individuals with Syndrome X have a "cluster" of symptoms that include high triglycerides and low HDL, high blood pressure, and some degree of glucose intolerance (inability to move glucose into the fat and muscle cells). In addition, after eating a meal they have high triglycerides levels that last throughout the day. They also have an increase in small, dense LDL (really, really bad LDL-cholesterol levels), and high plasminogen activator-1 levels, which means they are at higher risk for clotting.

What do the lab tests look like in a patient with Syndrome X? Fasting glucose is usually between 110 and 126, which is called impaired fasting glucose, or blood glucose between 140 and 200 two hours after drinking a glucose load during a glucose tolerance test. Fasting triglycerides levels are above 200 mg/dL, which usually accompanies low HDL cholesterol under 40 mg/dL. Some new information suggests that triglycerides levels below 150 mg/dL are associated with the small, dense LDL-cholesterol and may be a better number to strive for.

What's the bottom line here? These folks are at higher risk for heart attacks, period.

I

125

Intestines and absorption. The small intestine is a coiled tube, extending from the stomach to the ileocecal valve, where it joins the large intestine. Its average length in the living adult is 5 meters, approximately 16 ½ feet. However, it elongates after death, owing to the loss of muscle tone. In an interesting postmortem study of 109 adult subjects, it ranged from 3.35 – 7.16 meters in women and 4.88-7.85 meters in men, the average being 5.92 meters in females and 6.37 meters in males. Length was correlated with the height of the individual, but was independent of age. The large intestine is approximately 2 meters or 6 ½ feet. The total surface area of the intestines is more than 100 feet, or five times the area of the body's skin. The intestines process, at about one inch per minute, *40 tons*, of food over the course of 70 years.

Iron absorption. In order to absorb iron from food it is best to serve the iron-containing foods (such as prunes) with meat or a food high in vitamin C. Meat increases the acidity of the gastric juice and iron is absorbed better in a more acidic environment, while vitamin C changes the iron from ferric iron to ferrous iron, a more easily absorbed form.

Also, taking iron supplements with a food rich in vitamin C increases the absorption of iron from the supplement.

Iron deficiency and cooking with iron. Cooking with iron can significantly increase iron in the foods you eat. This is especially true for foods with high acidity such as tomatoes. For example, one serving of spaghetti sauce normally has less than one milligram of iron, but when cooked in an iron pot that amount can increase six-fold. (Hint: you have to have enough strength to lift the iron skillet if you're going to be cooking with cast iron.)

Is this a piece of good news or would it be considered hazardous to your health? It would certainly be of benefit for those groups needing extra iron, and that includes growing kids and pregnant moms. But for men as well as older women who are not at risk for iron deficiency, it is not beneficial. In addition, there is a hereditary disease known as hemochromatosis, in which the body accumulates way too much iron. This can result in liver disease and other serious manifestations of iron overload.

An Ethiopian study recently confirmed the benefits of cooking with iron pots. In a February 27, 1999 *Lancet* study, researchers compared 195 children who ate food cooked in aluminum pots with 207 children whose food was cooked in iron pots. After one year, blood tests demonstrated that the iron-deficiency anemia rate decreased from 57-12% in the group using the iron pots but only from 55-39% in the aluminum pot group. The children whose families used iron pots also grew slightly more, and none experienced iron overload.

Iron deficiency and restless leg syndrome. It has been estimated that one-fourth of the patients with restless leg syndrome have an iron deficiency.

Iron deficiency and tea drinking. Can tea drinking cause iron deficiency anemia? Yes. Tea drinking reduces the absorption of iron from the GI tract. A study performed in Israel evaluated 122 infants, aged 6-12 months. The percentage of tea-drinking infants with iron-deficiency anemia was 32.6% compared to 3.5% for the non-tea drinkers. The tea drinkers had significantly lower hemoglobins as well. (*American J Clinical Nutrition 1985*; 41:1210)

Iron and multivitamins. When purchasing a multivitamin, men and postmenopausal females should choose one with an iron content of less than 10 mg per day. Why? Preliminary evidence shows that iron may oxidize LDL cholesterol in the arteries and increase the risk of heart disease. Men with high iron levels have a higher risk of heart disease than men with low levels of serum iron. Postmenopausal women have stopped losing iron via menstruation and therefore will also accumulate iron.

Irradiation and food safety. Irradiating food to kill bacteria and other pathogens was first recommended in 1904 and first tested in the 1920s and 1930s. This process has been approved in the United States for killing or inactivating bacteria, fungi, parasites, and other creepy, crawly critters in flour, grains, fruits, vegetables, spices, poultry, beef and pork. For example, irradiating chicken can destroy *Salmonella* and *Campylobacter jejuni,* as well as other chicken-borne pathogens. Irradiation is also used to rid pork of trichinosis, and to rid fruits, vegetables and grains of all sorts of critters and insects. Irradiation can also kill *E. Coli O157:H7.*

Before you become a radical food fascist and disclaim the benefits of irradiating food, consider the following numbers: Food-borne illness strikes between 6 million and 80 million Americans yearly. More than 9,000 people die every year from food-borne illnesses, most of whom are the very young and the very old. Irradiating food can prevent many of these illnesses and deaths.

Now, for some questions about food irradiation. Is this the same type of irradiation used in cancer patients to zap cancer cells? Is this type of irradiation safe and effective for foods to be consumed by humans of all ages? Is this type of irradiation being used for all of the foods that it has been approved for? The answers—yes, yes, no. And now, the explanations.

Yes, this is the exact same type of irradiation used to destroy cancer cells. This irradiation is capable of destroying pathogens that lurk on the outside and the inside of fresh or frozen meat and chicken, strawberries, dried spices and any other source of contaminated food. The irradiation will either destroy the genetic code of the pathogen, disrupt its cell membranes,or inactivate essential enzymes necessary for growth and reproduction.

Yes, this type of radiation is quite safe. It kills the unwanted pathogens, however, it does not make food radioactive, just as external radiation does not make a patient radioactive. Food radiation does not result in DNA mutations and create cancer-causing chemicals in food as some of the consumer naysayers proclaim. Radiation alters the chemistry of the food just about as much as if it were heated or sun-dried.

Numerous studies have been performed on the safety of irradiated foods. The U.S. Army has performed studies on three generations of mice, rats, and beagles with nary a mishap. These research subjects developed no more cancer or inherited diseases than their control counterparts that were chowing down on canned foods or frozen, nonirradiated foods. Human research has demonstrated similar results. In addition, many tertiary care centers have elected to serve irradiated foods to their most severely immunocompromised patients—those that are at high risk of infection, such as burn patients and recipients of organ transplants. In addition, nursing homes are also choosing to use irradiated foods in order to reduce the number of food-borne infections in their elderly residents.

In addition, numerous agencies and organizations throughout the world have endorsed irradiation as a completely safe and effective practice. These organizations include the World Health Organization, the American Medical Association, the American Public Health Association, and the most amazing one of all—our very own Food and Drug Administration, a historically cautious agency that requires approximately 10 bazillion studies and 20 bazillion pages of documentation.

If you know that the food you buy is free of contamination with disease-causing microbes, you prepare it on clean surfaces with clean utensils, and you then cook it to just the right temperature, you probably have no need to buy irradiated food. However, for the individual writing this blurb on irradiated food, who isn't as squeaky clean as all of that, or who needs to eat in a fast food restaurant on more than one occasion, irradiation can offer real benefits.

Does irradiated food cost more money? Of course it does...what kind of a question is *that*? A few extra pennies per pound provide a wise investment for anyone who has a compromised immune system, as well as for very young children and very old adults. For everyone else, including those who are currently reading this very informative section, it offers extra protection that will save you days of diarrhea and protect your health for future decades.

"A two-pound turkey and a fifty-pound cranberry. That's Thanksgiving dinner at Three-Mile Island." —Johnny Carson

---

Indian Spiced Tea
Makes 6 servings

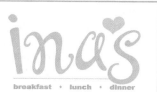

breakfast • lunch • dinner

6	Tbsp. Darjeerling Tea, loose
1/2	tsp. cardamom, dried
1/2	inch pc. cinnamon stick – broken into pieces
2	cloves, whole
6	cups water, just off the boil
	(Sugar and half and half are optional.)

Put tea, cardamom, cinnamon, cloves into a heated teapot.
Pour in water, cover and let steep for 4 minutes. Strain into cups.

Nutritional Info: One cup serving; Calories 4, Total fat 0 gr.; Protein 0.7gr.; Carbohydrates 0.1 gr.; Fiber 0 gr.; Sodium 9 mg.

Jammin'

Jam. Jam is a preparation of fruit cooked in a sugar syrup. The art of jam making began in the Middle East and was introduced into Europe by the Crusaders, who had discovered sugar cane and certain previously unknown fruits. A zillion fruits can be made into jam—bilberry jam, green tomato jam, pear jam, peach jam, apricot jam, strawberry jam, raspberry jam, toe jam (ha! Just checking to see if you're reading all of the jams), plum jam, redcurrant jam, rhubarb jam, watermelon jam, mango jam, haw jam, elderberry jam…ok, ok. You can add spices to enhance the flavor or you can add a little alcohol such as rum or Kirsch.

Marmalade and jam are one in the same, however, it appears as if there are two origins for the word marmalade. One states that it came from the Portuguese, *marmelo,* meaning jam. The second states that Joao Marmaloado (1450-1510) made the first breakfast "jam" by boiling oranges with sugar.

Jambalaya. A specialty of N'awlin's (New Orleans), inspired by Spanish paella and made of highly spiced rice, chicken, and ham. Various ingredients can be added; for example, sausage, peppers, tomatoes, prawns, or oysters

Jejunum. The jejunum is the middle portion of the small intestine, between the duodenum and the ileum. It is about 8 feet in length and comprises about two-fifths of the small intestine. It is derived from the word jejune, which means deficient or lacking in nutritive value. The jejunum was thought to be empty after death, hence the name.

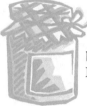

Jellies. Only fruits rich in pectin are suitable for making preserves, or jellies (apples, bilberry, redcurrants, mulberries, quinces, etc.). Vegetarians and vegans beware: Dessert jellies are made with gelatin or with calf's foot jelly.

Jellybeans. Jellybeans are bean-shaped, usually brightly colored candy with a hard sugar coating and a firm gelatinous filling. It has absolutely no nutritive value whatsoever, except that it is full of calories from the sugar.

JuicyFruit gum. What are the 4 predominant flavors in Juicy Fruit gum? Lemon, orange, pineapple, and banana.

Jujube. The jujube is an oval olive-size fruit with a smooth tough red skin, soft sweet yellowish or green flesh, and a hard seed in the middle. The jujube tree, which originated in China, along with its fruit, has been used medicinally for hundreds of years. The Far East countries export jujubes, either fresh or dried, also known as "red dates."

Junk foods. The *average* American gets one-fourth of their calories from junk foods. One third of all American adults get 50% of their calories from high-calorie, nutrient-poor foods like ice cream, cakes, cookies, candy, chips and soft drinks. More weight is gained as more junk food is consumed. Even though people who eat junk food get more calories, it doesn't mean that they get the appropriate nutrients. Most junk food junkies have lower blood levels of vitamins A, E, C, and B12, folate, and carotenoids. (*American Journal of Clinical Nutrition,* 72:929, 2000.)

Fruit Jam
Makes 2 pints

ina's
breakfast · lunch · dinner

    5   cups fruit (nectarines, peaches, apricots, plums)
         pitted and chopped
    2   Tbsp. lemon juice, fresh
    1   pkg. powdered fruit pectin *
 1-1/2   cups honey

In a heavy stainless steel pot, mix the fruit, lemon juice and pectin.

Stir over high heat and bring to a boil. (The fruit will give off a lot of liquid.) Stir in the honey.

Return to the boil and stir slowly for 5-6 minutes. When done, the mixture will look like thick syrup.

Cool. Pour into containers, cover and refrigerate.

*NOTE - You'll find the pectin in the baking section of the super-market.

Nutritional info: Serving size 1 Tablespoon: Calories 33; Total fat 0 gr.; Protein 0 gr.; Carbohydrates 9 gr.; Fiber 0 gr,; Sodium 2 mg.

J
131

is for...

Kiwi and Kuru

Kiwi fruit. Kiwi fruit is about the size of a large egg, with a greenish-brown rather hairy skin. The plant actually originated in China, but most of us associate the Kiwi fruit with "down under," New Zealand and Australia. It is also cultivated in California, western France and Israel. It is a rich source of vitamin C. Don't forget, Kiwi made the top ten list for the most powerful fruits.

Kava *(Piper methysticum).* Kava appears to be a natural remedy for anxiety and insomnia. It is made from the root of a perennial shrub native to the South Sea Islands and when taken in liquid form it provides a sense of euphoria and a sense of well-being. For this reason it was considered a sacred plant and it was used by the native islanders in just about every ritual imaginable—from celebrating the birth of an infant to paying homage to the death of a family or tribal member. It was used for wedding ceremonies, and as an "ice-breaker," so to speak, at parties.

In religious ceremonies, the tribal members chewed the kava root in order to prepare it for liquid consumption. Once chewed, it was spat into a bowl and mixed with coconut oil. Progress has been made in the preparation of kava, just in case you're interested. The root is now ground by mechanical means and the active ingredients, referred to as kavalactones, are extracted.

Kava appears to be quite promising as a modern-day anxiolytic. It should not be used in patients with depression and it may trigger an increased risk for suicide. Obviously, it should be used with caution and the patient population should be carefully screened before recommending it for use. Kava is best reserved for patients with situational anxiety who prefer an herbal approach versus a pharmaceutical approach. If used for anxiety, have the patient take the herb in the morning; if used for insomnia, have the patient take it in the evening. Advise the patients not to take it in addition to prescribed anxiolytics or sedatives or with alcohol.

KETCHUP

Ketchup. Two tablespoons of ketchup has 30 calories and 380 mg of sodium. It also contains 6 mg of the antioxidant lycopene. Lycopene has been touted as a powerful antioxidant with cardioprotective benefits and cancer prevention benefits. The problem with ketchup, however, is that in order to provide enough lycopene for the heart and cancer prevention benefits, you would have heart failure from the amount of sodium on board. Fast forward to the section on lycopane for better sources of this antioxidant. Our government has passed legislation that regulates the flow of ketchup. It has been mandated that ketchup must flow slower than 9 centimeters per 30 seconds or else the Ketchup Police will be down your throat in a heartbeat.

"Shake and shake
The catsup bottle,
None will come,
And then a lot'll."
—Richard Armour (1977)

KIDNEY STONES

Kidney stones. Until a few years ago, it was believed that too much calcium could aggravate or predispose individuals to kidney stones. Research from Harvard showed just the opposite. More calcium may actually prevent kidney stones by binding to oxalate, the main component of kidney stones, making oxalate unavailable to form stones. So, if you have kidney stones, can you safely drink milk? Yes. The calcium in the milk binds the oxalates. (Journal of the American Dietetic Association, March 1998.)

Kidney stones and women. Women who drink six or more 8-ounce servings of liquids a day have a 62% less risk of developing kidney stones than women who drink less. Caffeinated and decaf coffee, tea and wine were associated with less risk, while grapefruit juice increased the risk of kidney stones by 44%. Grapefruit juice may increase the risk because it creates a more alkaline urine or it may be an unexpected source of oxalate. The bottom line, drink tea or wine. Hold the grapefruit juice. (*Annals of Internal Medicine,* April 1998.)

Knorr. Carl Heinrich Knorr was a German industrialist who, after marrying his second wife in 1838, set up a small industrial plant for roasting coffee and chicory. You might wonder why he waited until he married his second wife. She had the money. Anyway, his business was profitable but didn't really take off until his two sons took over after his death. They expanded the business and began to manufacture pea, lentil, haricot beans, and sago flours, which were marketed in packets. These were the precursors of today's packet soups that you can find on your shelves of the grocery stores still bearing the family name, *Knorr.*

Kohlrabi. Ok, so I am trying to fill up the K chapter. It's a stretch, but it's also a cruciferous vegetable for you to add to your repertoire. Kohlrabi means "cabbage-turnip," and it belongs to the cabbage family. It's packed with fiber, vitamin C, iron, and potassium. In fact, one-half cup of kohlrabi has 16% more potassium than one-half cup of orange juice. So a bowl of kohlrabi in the morning to accompany your piece of whole grain toast and cup of coffee is a perfect way to start your day.

Kohlrabi, like the other cruciferous vegetables including cauliflower, Brussels sprouts, broccoli, and cabbage, contains natural cancer-fighting chemicals. These chemicals, known as isothiocyanates, assist in the inactivation and elimination of carcinogens.

Don't forget that all cruciferous vegetables contain goitrogens, substances that cause the thyroid gland to enlarge or develop a goiter. These goitrogens inhibit the ability of the thyroid gland to produce thyroid hormones which cause the thyroid to enlarge to compensate and produce more hormones. This does not pose a problem for healthy adults eating a healthy amount of cruciferous vegetables. However, individuals with an established thyroid problem or who are taking thyroid medications should be cognizant of this interaction.

Krauts. An American slur on Germans, taken from their love of sauerkraut.

Kuru (koo'roo). Kuru is a rapidly progressive neurological disease that is invariably fatal. The disease affects mostly adult women and children of both sexes belonging to the Fore (FOR-ae) tribe of New Guinea. Kuru is transmitted by the practice of ingesting tissue from an infected loved one who has died (ritual cannibalism) and rubbing infected tissues over the bodies of the women and children kin to the victim. The men of the Fore tribe rarely ate the dead and if they did partake, it would only be the red meat. The women and children however, ate everything from the liver to the small intestines to the heart. In fact, even the feces would be eaten, mixed with plants and cooked in banana leaves. If the dead loved one were a man, his penis, considered a rare delicacy, would be delivered with great care to the wife for consumption. A dying member of the Fore tribe would bequeath various body parts to their favorite kin in advance. "Their bellies are their cemeteries," remarked one of the observers of the Fore tribe. In fact, "I eat you" was a Fore greeting. That might have made me a bit nervous if I happened to be an anthropologist in New Guinea in the 1940s and 1950s.

As this practice continued, more and more Fore women were dying of a fatal disease known as kuru. Kuru meant shivering—with cold or with fear—and by 1950 kuru was killing women in every Fore village. Once the shivering began the women progressed through a series of neurologic symptoms primarily consisting of gait problems and mental decline. They eventually lost their ability to walk and swallow and they died of complications due to pneumonia and dementia. The flesh of those who died early of pneumonia was considered especially delicious, and was eaten by the children and other members of the family. Thus, the disease was passed from family member to family member.

The good news. The Fore tribe of New Guinea no longer practices cannibalism. So, the incidence of kuru has fallen dramatically and is nonexistent at this time.

"For what we are about to receive,
Oh Lord, 'tis Thee we thank,'
Said the cannibal as he cut a slice
Of the missionary's shank.
—E.Y. Harburg (1898-1981)

Kumquat. The kumquat is a citrus fruit originally from China and now cultivated in the Far East, Australia and the United States. It resembles a small orange, the size of a quail's egg, and has a sweet rind and a sour flesh. It is packed with vitamin A, potassium and calcium. Goooooood for ya', my little kumquat.

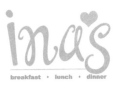

Kale stir-fried with Ginger
Makes 1 serving

breakfast · lunch · dinner

1	Tbsp.ginger root, fresh – peeled and minced
1/2	Tbsp. safflower or canola oil
1/4	lb. kale – coarsely chopped
1	tsp. soy sauce – reduced sodium
1/4	cup water

In a medium skillet, heat the oil and add the ginger. Stir over medium heat for about a minute.

Add the kale and raise the heat to medium/high.

Add the soy sauce and water and stir until the kale is a bit wilted but still slightly crunchy – about 3-4 minutes.

Serve warm or cold.

Nutritional Info: 1 serving: Calories 124; Total fat 7 gr.; Protein 3 gr.; Carbohydrates 11gr.; Fiber 7 gr.; Sodium 396 mg.

Lemons, Limeys and Lima Beans

Lemons. Light up a lemon. Researchers at Duke University are substituting citric acid derived from lemons for nicotine. Apparently citric acid mimics the sensations of smoking and patients find this a comparable substitute.

Lactose. Lactose is the naturally-occurring sugar found in milk.

Lactose intolerance. Approximately 25% of the U.S. adult population is unable to digest lactose, the main carbohydrate found in milk. In its pure form, lactose cannot be absorbed in the small bowel without the enzyme lactase. Lactase hydrolyzes lactose into two sugars, free glucose and galactose, both of which are absorbed rapidly and completely via the normal small intestine. The rate of lactase synthesis is high from birth until the age of five.

Between the ages of 5-14, many people have a genetically programmed reduction in the ability to produce the enzyme lactase, resulting in only 5-15% of the enzyme activity they had in the first five years. So, we obviously "grow" into this deficiency, and we're much more likely to do so depending on our genes. Only about 25% of the world's population is able to maintain a high degree of lactase activity throughout their adult life. If you have your full genetic complement of lactase as an adult you are referred to as having lactase persistence. If you are an individual with lactase nonpersistence, your levels of lactase are less than 10% of infantile levels.

The prevalence of lactase nonpersistence is higher in persons of African, Asian, Middle Eastern, Mediterranean, and Native American ancestry. In contrast, only about 5% of individuals with Northern European ancestors and 15% of those with central European ancestors are nonpersistent. So, when considering the diagnosis of lactose intolerance, consider the genes.

Many Americans have self-diagnosed lactose intolerance because of the media hype surrounding this condition. As a result, this population of self-diagnosed individuals is missing out on one of the best sources of vitamin D and calcium, as well as other essential proteins provided by milk and milk products.

Most of the individuals who are self-diagnosed can absorb lactose without any problems. And, new research suggests that individuals who have been definitively diagnosed with lactose intolerance may be able to tolerate moderate amounts of the carbohydrate. The key is to initially consume very small amounts of lactose. Start with one-half to one cup of milk with meals, and slowly increase the amount to one to two cups daily in two or three divided doses. If milk is consumed regularly, the bacteria in the large intestines can adapt and metabolize lactose.

FYI—Yogurt (8 oz.) contains 300-400 mg of calcium and 10-15 grams of lactose. Eight ounces of milk contains 290-300 mg of calcium and 10-12 grams of lactose. Ice cream (4 oz.) contains 80 mg of calcium and 4.5-5.0 grams of lactose. Hard cheese (1 oz) contains 150-275 mg of calcium and only 0-1 mg of lactose. (*Environmental Nutrition*, December 1997; *Patient Care;* April 15, 1997.)

Lead. Lead poisoning is much more common in infants and children for various reasons. First, the blood-brain barrier is immature prior to the age of three, allowing lead to enter the brain more readily. Second, ingested lead has a 40% bioavailability in children as compared to a 10% bioavailability in adults. Third, childhood behaviors associated with frequent hand-to-mouth gestures greatly increase the risk of lead ingestion. The recommended lead levels are less than 10 micrograms per deciliter (10 mg/dL). The Agency for Toxic Substances and disease registry estimates that approximately 17% of the U.S. preschool children have abnormally high levels of lead exceeding 15 mg/dL.

Serum lead levels once thought to be safe have been shown to be associated with IQ deficits, behavior disorders, slowed growth and impaired hearing. The impairment of cognitive function begins at levels greater than 10 mg/dL, even though clinical symptoms are not apparent. Sources of exposure include lead-based paint (inner city housing and old homes), soil and dust (near the old house with falling paint chips), tap water (hot tap water from old homes with lead solder on pipe connections), occupational and recreational exposures (furniture refinishing, stained-glass, or pottery making), airborne exposures (near smelters or near battery-manufacturing plants), and dishware and canned foods.

Most china, porcelain, earthenware and crystal contain varying amounts of lead used during the manufacturing process. However, when properly fired during manufacturing the dishes are not considered to be dangerous. Regulations vary from country to country, however, the U.S., Japan, and Great Britain have the strictest regulations on lead content. One important point to remember—after years of use, lead may leach out of the china, porcelain or crystal container. Avoid storing food or drink in these containers for long periods of time. If you desire to serve wine in a crystal decanter, this is perfectly safe and lovely. But, don't store the wine in the decanter—either drink it all or pour it back in the original bottle. (NOTE: If you have to screw off the top of the wine bottle you don't need to decant it.) Imported food products may also be contaminated by lead used to solder cans. Foreign countries do not have to adhere to U.S. restrictions, so your refried beans from Mexico might be laced with lead.

Diets low in calcium, iron and possibly protein increase the body's absorption and retention of lead, while a diet replete with these nutrients protects against lead build-up.

LEFTOVERS

L

141

Leftovers. Contrary to popular belief, do no let leftovers cool before you refrigerate them. You are just inviting bacteria to multiply if the food cools down below 140° F. The bugs continue to multiply until food has cooled below 40° F. The danger zone then, appears to be between 40° F and 140° F. So, get those leftovers into the refrigerator as soon as possible and don't worry about heating up the refrigerator with warm food! Put the

HISTORICAL HIGHLIGHT

In the 1500s, a big kettle was used for cooking. Every day they lit a fire and added vegetables to the pot with just a bit of meat. They would eat the stew or porridge for dinner, leaving leftovers in the pot to get cold overnight. The process would start all over again the next morning by adding more vegetables and small portions of meat. The stew could stay in the pot for days on end, spawning the rhyme, "Peas porridge hot, peas porridge cold, peas porridge in the pot, nine days old."

leftovers in shallow containers to help the foods cool down as quickly as possible. In fact, if your freezer has a bit of room, throw the leftovers in the freezer temporarily to cool the leftovers faster. (*Environmental Nutrition*, September 2000.)

"Some people do wonderful things with leftovers —
they throw them out." –Anonymous

Legumes. Legumes (dried beans, dried peas, lentils and peanuts) all qualify as heart-healthy and colon-healthy proteins. The B vitamin folate, the insoluble fiber, and the top quality and quantity of protein all make legumes a food source not to be missed. Beans are also very low in sodium, unless you consume your beans out of a can. Canned beans have as much as 400 mg per half-cup, however, rinsing canned beans under cold water may reduce the sodium content by as much as 40%.

Leptin. Leptin is a chemical produced by fat cells in the body. Its major role in life is to signal the brain that we have enough fat cells and that we can stop eating. Obviously, it doesn't seem to work in most of us. Genetically altered mice that lack the leptin gene become obese. They lack the leptin signal to stop eating, so it's a feeding frenzy from the get-go.

The leptin molecule may also be the signal for puberty. Preliminary studies have shown that when the researchers inject young prepubescent mice with leptin, the young ladies reach sexual maturity much earlier than their giggly prepubescent friends who have only received a saline injection. This makes the leptin molecule a prime suspect as the principal initiator of puberty and links previously published data that ties the amount of fat cells to the onset of puberty in young girls. Rose E. Frisch and colleagues at the Harvard School of Public Health published the first paper showing that a critical amount of fat was necessary for puberty and continued ovulation. This landmark study was quite controversial back in 1974 when it was first published. Since that time over 100 studies have been published on the subject. Evidence continues to build supporting the fat/leptin/puberty hypothesis in young girls. The verdict is still out on what triggers the onset of puberty in the male.

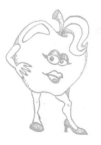

Licorice root (*Glycyrrhiza glabra* or "sweet and smooth root"). Licorice root has been used for medicinal purposes and for flavoring foods for millenniums, around three millenniums to be exact. The Greeks, Egyptians, and Chinese worshipped this root. It is 50 times sweeter than sugar and is capable of masking pungent tastes in medicines and is therefore used as a flavoring in cough syrups, throat lozenges, gum, candy, and tobacco. In fact, 90% of the licorice used in the United States is used to flavor tobacco products like cigarettes and chewing tobacco. Most of the "licorice" candies, including Twizzlers (the red ones), Good n' Plenty, and black jelly beans in the United States are flavored with anise, not natural licorice. (Black Twizzlers contain natural licorice root extract in combination with anise oil.)

You might wonder why our candies in the U.S. contain mostly anise instead of the natural licorice root. Our Food and Drug Administration allows candy to contain up to 3% natural licorice by weight, but most contain no more than 2%, or about 0.5 gm in four twisted "ropes" of Twizzlers. In Europe, it's a different story. Black licorice, candy and cough drops contain from 5% to 65% natural licorice.

Two sticks of European black licorice per day for seven days may result in a weight gain of one to five pounds. The main active ingredient of licorice is glycyrrhizin or glycyrrhetic acid and has a chemical structure similar to aldosterone, the adrenal hormone responsible for sodium and water retention. This retention can lead to hypertension with headaches, vomiting, and photophobia. This has also been referred to as Halloween Hypertension, and is primarily seen in children during the week or two after Halloween. The physical assessment clue is a black tongue.☺ If natural licorice is taken for long periods of time the sodium retention can result in potassium loss through the kidneys. Natural licorice in any form is not recommended for individuals with high blood pressure, heart disease, and diabetes or for pregnant or lactating women.

Why would you take licorice root as an alternative therapy? As a medicinal herb, licorice has been used to soothe irritated stomachs, squelch irritating coughs, and as an expectorant. Herbalists in Europe and the U.S. also use licorice root to treat stomach and duodenal ulcers and to treat adrenal insufficiency. Flavonoids, anti-inflammatory compounds, are also present in licorice root and may be responsible for soothing the lining of the upper GI tract and suppressing the cough reflex.

How much licorice should you take? Read all labels on any products before taking a slug of it for your cough. The recommended daily dose is 5-15 grams of the dried root made into a tea. Do not take for longer than 4-6 weeks. Read the label, read the label, read the label.

Don't forget that black licorice candy from Europe can be hazardous to your blood pressure and your heart when taken in mega-amounts.

Lima beans. It's not often that one happens upon a lima bean recipe. So, here's one to tempt the taste buds:

Sauté 1 chopped tomato and 3 diced garlic cloves in 2 Tbs. of olive oil. Add 2 cups of frozen lima beans and stir until heated through. Toss in 1 Tbs. of chopped parsley, 2 Tbs. of red wine vinegar, and salt and pepper to taste.

Limey. Limey is an American slang expression for British sailors, who regularly consumed lemons and limes and other citrus fruits to prevent scurvy on their long ocean voyages. This is somewhat of a misnomer, however, because truth be told, the lemon is better equipped to protect from scurvy (vitamin C deficiency) than the lime. Lime juice has a lower vitamin C content than lemon juice and it appears that the vitamin C molecule is much less stable in lime juice than in lemon juice.

Full credit for this discovery of the relationship of vitamin C to scurvy is given to Dr. James Lind, a British ship's surgeon who is credited with the first controlled clinical study in the history of medicine. On May 20, 1747, Dr. Lind examined 12 sailors on board ship with signs and symptoms of scurvy. He described the sailors as having "putrid gums, the spots and lassitude, with the weakness of the knees." They were divided into six groups, two sailors per group. One of the groups was given two oranges and one lemon per day, which he said, "They ate with greediness." By the end of six days one of the two was ready to return to duty as a sailor and by the end of the trip (June 16, 1747) both sailors in the fruit group had sufficiently recovered. In fact the second sailor to recover was appointed as the nurse to the other patients. The other five groups received various combinations of other concoctions (including cider, wine, puddings, boiled biscuits with sugar and mutton-broth) but they did not receive fresh fruit. None of the other men in the other groups recovered from their scurvy.

"There's no danger of my getting scurvy [while in England], as I have to consume at least two gin-and-limes every evening to keep the cold out."
—SJ Perelman (1904-1979.)

Lush. Dr. Thomas Lushington (1590-1661) has the distinction of having his name shortened to lush…the term fondly used for an individual who enjoys a little too much fruit of the vine. Dr. Lushington was an English chaplain known for his fondness for liquor. The term lush was actually originally used as a slang term for beer, but has evolved into the slang term for a drunkard.

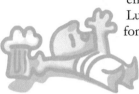

LYCOPENE

Lycopene. Lycopene is a powerful antioxidant (twice as powerful as beta carotene) that does most of its work preventing cancers below the belt—colon, prostate and cervical. Lycopene belongs to the family of carotenoids that give vegetables and fruits their vibrant colors. This carotenoid just so happens to give tomatoes their lusciously deep red color. Other vegetables that contain lycopene include pink grapefruit, watermelon and guava.

In order for the lycopene to exert its powerful effects the tomatoes should be cooked. Cooking breaks down the cell walls in tomatoes and unleashes the effects of lycopene. By cooking the tomatoes in a little olive oil, lycopene will be absorbed even further, because it is fat-soluble.

So what is your best bet for adding lycopene to your diet? Tomato sauces top the list with 23 mg of lycopene per ½ cup serving. Salsa is at the bottom of the list with 3 mg per 2 tablespoons and canned tomatoes sit right in the middle with 11 mg per ½ cup. (*Environmental Nutrition*, March 1999)

Everything you have ever wanted to know about lycopene can be found at www.lycopene.com. It's chock-full of research findings, recipes for prostate-healthy eating, and of course, none other than the H.J. Heinz Company sponsors it.

Lemon Cooler
Makes 4 servings

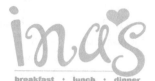

1 cup lemon juice, fresh (about 6 lemons) – divided in half
2 cups ice water
2 cups ice, crushed – divided in half
1/2 cup sugar, superfine – divided in half

Into a blender put 1/2 cup lemon juice, 1 cup of ice water, 1 cup of crushed ice and 1/4 cup sugar. Blend on high speed until frothy.

Pour into a pitcher and repeat with the remaining ingredients.

Nutritional info: For 1 serving: Calories 112; Total fat 0 gr.; Protein 0.2 gr.; Carbohydrates 30 gr.; Fiber 0.2 gr.; Sodium 5 mg.

M

is for...

Mad Cows and
Big Macs

Mad cow disease. This devastating neurological deterioration is fatal in all cases—whether you are a sheep, a cow, a cannibal, or a human with non-cannibalistic preferences. In sheep the disease is known as scrapie (SCRAY-pee), in cows it is known as bovine spongiform encephalopathy (BSE), in the Fore cannibal tribe of New Guinea it is known as kuru, and in non-cannibalistic humans it is referred to as Creutzfeldt-Jakob disease (CJD) or *variant* Creutzfeldt-Jakob disease (vCJD).

The first cases of "mad cow" disease appeared in Britain in 1987. Cows were observed to be disoriented, irritable, apprehensive and unable to stand or walk without a staggering, unsteady gait. Autopsies on the bovine brain revealed "spongy" areas and the name bovine spongiform encephalopathy was given to this disease in cattle. The autopsy findings were similar to those seen in humans dying of CJD and in sheep dying of scrapie. (The term scrapie originates from the behavior of sheep with this illness. The disoriented, demented sheep stand next to the barn or fence and scrape their flank against it until it bleeds.)

In 1996, the first ten British citizens were diagnosed with "mad cow" disease. Since their brain tissue resembled that of the mad cows and that of humans dying of CJD, the British pathologists named it *variant* CJD (vCJD). Since 1996, over 85 British citizens have died from vCJD and over 100 have died throughout the European nations. Italy, Germany, France, Spain, Ireland, Belgium, Denmark, Luxembourg, the Netherlands, Switzerland, and Liechtenstein (Where the hell is Liechtenstein?) have all reported cattle infected with mad cow disease.

The cause of BSE is a mutant prion (PREE-on). This is not a virus, parasite, bacteria, fungus, or any other type of known infectious agent. The brains of all mammals (and that includes us, humans) contain structural proteins in the brain known as prions. An unknown trigger causes the prion to undergo a structural "unfolding," which in turn acts as a toxin causing the surrounding brain tissue to degenerate. Once the prion unfolds, the damage to neighboring tissue results in a progressive, unremitting, and rapid deterioration of mental and motor function.

The exact trigger for the unfolding of the prion is unknown, however, it is most likely triggered by eating brain or spinal cord tissue from another infected animal. Eating cattle infected with the mutant prion causes the vCJD in Europe. The cattle were infected by eating rendered meat-and-bone meal protein supplements made from sheep, cows, pigs, poultry, road kill, and any other dead animal that happened upon the rendering machine. (Rendering, by the way, means to boil and grind up carcasses of dead animals—including bones, brains, spinal cords, and internal organs.) Most likely the culprit was from renderings of sheep with scrapie and other cattle with BSE.

Notice that the list of countries mentioned earlier did *not* include the U.S. No cases of infected cattle or human forms of vCJD have been diagnosed in the U.S. and hopefully it will stay that way. Our FDA, USDA, and every other regulating agency have their hands in the pot on this one, and safeguards have been put into place. First of all, the USDA banned the importation of sheep and goats to the U.S. as far back as 1950 after a flock of British sheep were reported to have scrapie. They also banned their rumination by-products. The importation of cattle from England was banned in 1989. Fewer than 500 cows from the British Isles made it across the Atlantic Ocean in the 1980s. Of those 500, only 32 entered the food chain. The chance that even one cow was infected is one in 10 billion.

Secondly, the FDA has prohibited animal-feed mills from mixing meat-and-bone meal made from rendered cows and sheep into feed for cows and sheep. The supplements can be fed to swine and poultry, however, because they do not get BSE-like illnesses from food.

The third reason it will be tough for BSE to make its way into our food chain is because of good old McDonald's. Even though they are killing us with the fries and burgers in one way or another, they are adamant that their hamburger source is free of contamination. And, when McDonald's talks, *everyone* listens. McDonald's rules the roost when it comes to beef sales throughout the world. If Mickey D's says that all cattle used for its all-beef patties should have documentation that they have not been fed meat-and-bonemeal made from cows and sheep, then by cracky, it's a mandate.

Lastly, the beef industry stopped using stun guns to prepare cattle for the slaughterhouse. The explosive blast from the stun gun blew brain tissue throughout the carcass, causing a potential route of infection with prions in nervous system tissue. In cows with BSE, brain tissue is highly infectious.

Hmmmm, you say. If people didn't eat cow brains or spinal cords, how did they acquire this illness? Most likely from eating inexpensive beef products that contained mechanically separated meat. This type of meat is a paste produced by compressing carcasses. This paste may have contained spinal cords, and was used in preparing hot dogs, sausages, and burgers. Do we use mechanically separated meat in the U.S.? Yes, but rarely. And, the label on the package must state that it includes mechanically separated beef. Unfortunately, there are no labels on hot dogs purchased from hot dog stands or sausages as a side order at you favorite breakfast establishment.

So, is a filet mignon safe? Yes. How about a good old hot dog at Wrigley Field? Yes. How about a good old hot dog in jolly old England? Well, not exactly. The European Union has banned mechanically separated beef and that ban should be in full effect by the end of 2001.

Can vegetarians acquire vCJD? Yes, and they have. Most likely their exposure was through milk, or gelatin which is made from beef. Or, vCJD may incubate for decades (the incubation period is unknown at this time), and the vegetarian may have eaten infected beef in the years prior to becoming a vegetarian.

What are the safest cuts of meat? Boneless steaks such as filet mignon, roasts, or other whole cuts of beef are the safest. T-bone, porterhouse, standing rib roast, prime rib with bone, and bone-in chuck blade roast may contain spinal cord tissue or small groups of nerves that line the spinal cord known as dorsal root ganglia, which are infectious if they come from an infected cow. For more information on these neurological diseases see Appendix B.

> **FACT:** In January 2001 the USDA recommended that anyone who had lived in France, Portugal, or Ireland for a total of 10 years since 1980 be prohibited from donating blood. The year before, the USDA recommended a similar exclusion for anyone living in Britain for six months between 1980 and 1996. The interesting point to the blood donor recommendation is that there is absolutely *no* evidence that the disease can be transmitted through a blood transfusion in the first place. Better to be safe than sorry, I suppose.

MACADAMIA

Macadamia nuts. John MacAdam M.D., was a Scottish physician who relocated to Australia circa 1855 to teach and practice medicine. He befriended a botanist after his move—a gentlemen by the name of Ferdinand von Mueller. Von Mueller was exploring the outback of Australia one fine day in 1857 when he happened upon what he thought was an entirely new species of tree that produced a fascinating nut. He was intrigued by his finding and reviewed the world's botanical literature to determine whether or not this tree existed in the world of botany at the time. He determined that it was a new find, and he named the nut of the tree after his physician and friend, John MacAdam.

Macular degeneration. Age-related macular degeneration (AMD) is a common cause of impaired vision in older adults. It occurs when the cells in the central part of the retina, called the macula, degenerate, slowly resulting in blurred central vision. When this occurs it is difficult for the patient to drive, read, and perform other activities that require central vision. Most macular degeneration is referred to as "dry" AMD. A rare form of macular degeneration is known as "wet" age-related macular degeneration. This occurs when abnormal blood vessels grow in the retina and start to leak blood and serum into the back of the eye. This can result in a sudden deterioration of vision.

How can this be prevented or delayed? Go straight to the produce counter and stock up on those "green leafys," especially spinach, kale, broccoli, and collard greens. These contain certain antioxidants (lutein and zeaxanthin) and may reduce the incidence of age-related macular degeneration by as much as 43%. Next stop—the seafood counter. Stock up on the fish that contain the highest amounts of omega-3 fatty acids. A study in the March 2000 *Archives of Ophthalmology* found that older adults who ate fish more than once a week had only half the risk of late-stage AMD as those who ate it less than once a month. Third stop—the vitamin and dietary supplement section of the grocery store. Vitamin C and vitamin E, the antioxidant vitamins, may reduce the risk of developing AMD. The verdict is still out on these vitamin supplements for this use, but they're important for other reasons, so grab a couple of bottles. Last stop—look in the B section of the dietary supplements and consider buying the herb, bilberry. Preliminary studies suggest that bilberry extract may halt the progression of cataracts as well as AMD. (*Dr. Andrew Weil's Self Healing*, March 2001.)

NOTE: The "wet" form of AMD is due to bleeding under the retina. Avoid any nutrients or dietary supplements that predispose to bleeding, including garlic, gingko, ginger, glucosamine and large doses of vitamin E. Each of these dietary supplements inhibits platelet aggregation and predisposes the individual to bleeding.

Magnesium. Women need 310 mg per day for ages 19 through 30 or 320 mg per day over age 30; men need 400 mg per day for ages 19 through 30, or 420 mg per day over age 30; the upper limit from supplements alone should not exceed 350 mg/day. The total amount of magnesium from supplements and diet should not exceed 700 mg per day.

Research suggests that a magnesium deficiency may increase the risk of diabetes, high blood pressure, heart disease, osteoporosis and migraines. For starters, the average American doesn't consume enough magnesium to replace what they are losing through the urine on a daily basis. The biggest reason for the under-consumption is that magnesium is found in the foods that most Americans do not consume in adequate amounts. This includes leafy green vegetables, whole grains, beans and nuts. In other words, French fries and hamburgers supply miniscule amounts of magnesium, even on a good day.

Magnesium and diabetes. Magnesium is required for the secretion of insulin from the pancreas. Without enough magnesium the pancreas will fail to secrete the needed amount to control blood glucose levels. Insulin becomes ineffective, the patient becomes less insulin sensitive, and the trek toward the development of type 2 diabetes has begun. Two large studies have demonstrated a relationship between low magnesium levels and the progression to type 2 diabetes. Does this mean that taking magnesium supplements will lower blood sugar in the diabetic? No, not at this time. However, magnesium might *prevent* diabetes, so just to play the prevention game, make sure you get the RDA of 400 mg from food and, if necessary, a supplement. (*American Journal of Clinical Nutrition,* 55: 1992; 1018. and *The Journal of Clinical Epidemiology,* 48: 1995; 927.)

M
151

Magnesium and migraines. A small number of women who suffer from migraine headaches may be deficient in magnesium. In one of two small studies, patients who took 600 mg of magnesium a day for 12 weeks went from three attacks per month to two. That might not sound like a lot, however, if you are the one with debilitating migraine headaches this reduction may be a lifesaver. (*Cephalgia* 16; 257, 1996).

Magnesium and osteoporosis. It appears as if magnesium may be important for strong bones and for the prevention of osteoporosis. Choosing a calcium supplement with magnesium may give an added boost for bone protection.

M & M's. One of the biggest sellers for the Mars Company is M & M's. The average number of M & M's per standard package is 57, give or take one or two. Of that number, 33% are dark brown, 25% are yellow, 19% are orange, 14% are blue, and 9% are green. Since the green M & M's have the folk lore reputation of being a powerful aphrodisiac, one wonders if the Mars Company hasn't lost its libido. Each M & M has 4.2 calories.

In 1976 the Mars Company took red M & M's off the market, responding to the mass hysteria triggered by the media. The media hyped the fact that red M & M's were made with the carcinogenic red dye number 2. This wasn't true, red dye number 2 was not used, however, the damage was already done. The teeming masses became so hysterical that it was the company's only recourse. Red M & M's have since been reintroduced to the market without the mass hysteria. Red M & M's are colored with red dye number 3, a noncarcinogenic chemical additive.

Margarine. Margarine or butter? Butter or margarine? Which one is better, butter? Well, neither of the above choices wins the contest for food of the day, week, or even year, for that matter. They are both full of the "bad" fats, although margarine might be considered the more ominous of the two, due to its "trans fats." Now, having said that, not all margarines are created equal in terms of trans fat content. As a general rule of thumb, the softer the margarine, the less trans fat it contains. So tub margarine is better for you than stick margarine. So grab a tub of soft margarine instead of a stick of margarine or a stick of butter. Oh boy. Just don't eat a lot of any of the above. Or, check the grocery shelves for the trans fat-free margarines.

Martini. The martini cocktail was invented in 1863 by a San Francisco bartender named Jerry Thomas (also credited for the Tom and Jerry). He purportedly named the drink after the town of Martinez upon learning that this was the destination of a departing customer.

Meat eater. Meat eater is a slang term for a policeman or politician who accepts or extorts bribes (graft). If you are not one of the above meat eaters, but do like a piece of meat on occasion you should consider choosing sirloin instead of prime rib. A trimmed16-ounce prime rib has 1,000 calories and two day's worth of saturated fat, however, a trimmed 12-ounce sirloin has only 400 calories and less than half a day's saturated fat.

Meat packer

HISTORICAL HIGHLIGHT

Perhaps the most famous of all meat packers in the world was Sam Wilson of Troy, New York. His nickname was *Uncle Sam* Wilson and he supplied meat to the troops of the War of 1812. The beef Wilson shipped out was stamped with the initials U.S. and although he intended the U.S. as an abbreviation for the United States, it also came to be identified with Wilson himself, or *Uncle Sam*. Cartoonists of the time portrayed him with a white goatee, dressed in a top hat and the patriotic colors of red, white and blue. In 1961 Congress made Uncle Sam official as the United States' "mascot" so to speak. A resolution recognized Sam Wilson, the meat packer from Troy, New York, as *Uncle Sam's* namesake.

M
153

Mediterranean diet. What is the Mediterranean-style diet? Well, if you have a history of heart disease or if you have already had a myocardial infarction (heart attack), you may want to listen up. The Mediterranean-style diet is rich in fruits, vegetables, whole grains, legumes, and fish with 30% of the calories from fat but only 8% of the fat calories as saturated fat. According to a study in the February 16, 1999 issue of the journal *Circulation,* patients with heart disease who followed the Mediterranean diet guidelines had a 50-70% lower risk of a second heart attack in the four years of follow-up as compared to the patients who followed the traditional western diet of 34% fat with 12% saturated fats. The authors of the study credit the omega-3 fatty acids found in the fish, nuts, canola oil and flaxseed as playing a major role in cardiac protection. If you need information on switching to a Mediterranean-style diet call your friendly nutritionist (1-800-366-1655) for a consultation.

Melatonin and tumor growth. Linoleic acid, the primary fat in corn oil, has been shown to stimulate the growth of tumors in rats, but only in the absence of melatonin, the hormone produced by the pineal gland at night. During the nighttime hours when an animal produces melatonin, tumor production of a growth chemical produced from linoleic acid decreased to negligible amounts. Cancer in these rats grew at roughly one-half the rate of the tumors in rats with their melatonin-producing pineal gland removed. Providing extra melatonin as a late-afternoon supplement was important—giving it early in the daytime had no effect.

Memory. Try this for a short-term memory boost: 1 large tart apple and a cup of cashew nuts blended until smooth and chilled. Spread a little on whole-wheat crackers and enjoy. Nibble on this while studying and it may help you remember what you are reading. (Alzheimer's Prevention Foundation, Dharma Singh Khalsa, MD, Tucson, AZ.)

M
154

Mercury. Mercury is a metal that accumulates in fish. Mercury excess is particularly dangerous for pregnant women since it can cause birth defects in the developing embryo. Various fish accumulate mercury in different amounts. Points are given for the type of fish consumed, with 10 points being the worst fish in terms of mercury contamination. Consuming more than 70 points per week can cause symptoms of mercury poisoning, including numbness in the extremities and diminished motor skills. The highest amounts of mercury are found in swordfish, fresh tuna, pike or walleye. In fact each of those receives 10 points for a one-ounce serving. Halibut gets 5 points on the scale and canned tuna, shrimp, crab, lobster, and salmon receive 2 points per one-ounce serving.

Milk. Nonfat dry milk can add a significant protein and calcium boost to foods, without adding fat or cholesterol. Simply mix the powder into casseroles, creamy soups, puddings, dressings, quick breads, pancakes, cookies, or shakes. One-third cup contains only 80 calories, yet provides 8 grams of protein and 300 mg of calcium, the same as in a cup of fluid milk.

| **FACT:** | A glass of milk may contain minute amounts of up to *80* different antibiotics. |

How do you coax a cow to produce more milk? A kick in the dairy air? No, not exactly. The 43rd International Science and Engineering Fair in Nashville shed some light on this dilemma. An eight-week study found that cows increased their production of milk by 6.2% if they listened to country music. Rock music only increased the output by 4.7%, and Mozart was a dismal failure—only a 1.6% increase in milk output with classical music.

"Happiness is seeing your mother-in-law's picture on the back of a milk carton." —Anonymous

Milk thistle. Andrew Weil, M.D. suggests taking milk thistle for at least two months after receiving chemotherapy. Milk thistle is a natural remedy that helps the liver to recover from toxins such as drugs. He suggests the brand name Thisilyn from Nature's Way. (Weil, A. *Self Healing.* January 2001.)

Miso. Miso is a fermented soybean paste made with salt and often with rice or barley. The lighter varieties tend to be milder, the darker colors are more flavorful. So, if you are looking to add a bit of soy to your diet, how about a cup of miso soup.

Multivitamins. Questions and Answers—the scoop.
Q. Should you buy generic multivitamins or should you fork out the big bucks for the expensive brands?
A. Generic multivitamins are just as effective as the more expensive brands, so unless you just enjoy being a "name dropper" and paying more money to have a brand name on the shelf, buy the less expensive stuff.

Q. Some of the multivitamins say they contain sugar and starch additives. Should I shun those in favor of multivitamins that don't have those "fillers"?

A. No. Don't shun the sugar and starch additives as they help with the absorption of the contents of the multivitamins; they are not just "fillers." However, do ignore the hype about special features such as "extended release," "time-release," etc. There is no optimal time to absorb nutrients. Therefore, having vitamins available throughout the day is of little value. An exception to the rule is nicotinic acid, or niacin. This B vitamin is sometimes prescribed in the time-release form to avoid the uncomfortable side effect of flushing, however, this form is actually *more* toxic to the liver.

To improve absorbability, take your supplement with food. "Chelated" vitamins supposedly offer superior absorption. However, a chelated nutrient breaks down as soon as it hits the acid-rich stomach and is absorbed just like other nutrients. Do not take vitamins with coffee, since the acid can cancel out some of the nutrients.

Q. Should you buy the natural form or the synthetic form of the vitamin?

A. Synthetic vitamins are just fine *except* for vitamin E, which is more potent in the natural form. How do you know if vitamin E is natural or synthetic? Flip the bottle of vitamin E on its side and read the small print. The contents will be described as dl-alpha tocopherol or d-alpha tocopherol. The d form of alpha tocopherol is the *natural* form of the vitamin and is the more potent form.

If perchance, you have synthetic on your kitchen shelf, don't toss it in the trash. Finish using the bottle that you have but adjust the dose accordingly. If 200 IU is recommended in the natural form of the vitamin use 300-400 IU of the synthetic form. If 400 IU is recommended in the natural form of vitamin E, use 500-600 IU of the synthetic form.

Close to 30% of U.S. adults have low serum levels of vitamin E, according to the Centers for Disease Control. Of all the groups studied, African-Americans had the lowest concentrations. Individuals deficient in this vitamin, which is best obtained from supplements, as mentioned, may be at increased risk for heart disease and cancer. (*American Journal of Epidemiology*, August 1999)

Folic acid and vitamin B12 are better absorbed as supplements. The natural form of folic acid, folate, is not absorbed well from foods (even from good sources like spinach, orange juice, and beans), making a supplement a good idea. Besides a multivitamin providing plenty of folic acid (at least 400 micrograms or 0.4 mg), the U.S government also now mandates that all "enriched" grains contain folic acid. The same is true for B12. A B12 supplement is better absorbed than foods containing B12.

Q. How many vitamins and minerals should be included in a "multivitamin?"

A. Look for at least 20. Several "key" nutrients fall short in the American diet and should be included *for sure* in a multivitamin. These include vitamin D (especially if you are over 50 and trying to protect your bones), B12, folate, calcium, copper, iron, magnesium, selenium, and zinc.

NOTE: The DV for iron is 18 mg for premenopausal women in order to replace the amount lost with menstruation; but 0 mg for men and postmenopausal women. High amounts of iron act as an oxidant on LDL-cholesterol. Oxidation of LDL-cholesterol results in plaque formation in the arteries with resultant atherosclerosis.

Q. What is the RDA or DV?

A. Nutritionists have traditionally used the RDA (Recommended Daily Allowance) to provide information on the amount of vitamin or mineral needed daily in order to prevent a nutritional deficiency. The DV (Daily Value) is a variation on that theme and a recent name change to take the place of RDA. These amounts are calculated with an added margin for protection, so anything more than 100% is *not* necessary except in strict vegetarians, individuals on restricted weight loss diets, or the elderly.

The amounts listed on the side of the multivitamin are *not* therapeutic doses of vitamins. In other words, 60 IUs (international units) of vitamin E is not considered to be a useful "antioxidant" dose, however it *is* considered to be enough of a dose to prevent any complications from vitamin E deficiency. If an individual is consuming vitamin E for its purported therapeutic antioxidant effects, the daily dose ranges between 100 IU to 800 IU. This would of course mean that an additional dose of vitamin E would have to be consumed in order to fulfill the therapeutic requirement.

M
157

Q. Should I buy a vitamin that has a USP designation on it?

A. The USP on the label indicates that a supplement meets five quality standards set by the United States Pharmacopoeia for vitamin, mineral, botanical and herbal supplements: 1) disintegration, 2) dissolution, 3) potency, 4) purity and 5) expiration date. Don't be impressed with a label that only advertises "laboratory tested" or "quality assured." This means little without a USP label.

Q. What does fat-soluble versus water-soluble mean?

A. Vitamins A, D, E, and K are fat-soluble vitamins, which means that they are attached to lipids in the blood. To reap the necessary benefits of fat-soluble vitamins, you need to have some fat in your diet. The body can store excess amounts of fat-soluble vitamins.

The B vitamins and vitamin C are water-soluble, which cleverly means they dissolve in water. Most are not stored in the body and excess vitamins are excreted via the kidneys. However, taken in "mega-doses," these water-soluble vitamins can be toxic. For example, the body can only retain 500 mg of vitamin C at one time. The kidneys will immediately excrete a dose greater 500 mg. So, your toilet will reap the benefits of a 1,000 mg dose of vitamin C, you will not.

The "anti-oxidant" dose of vitamin C is 200 mg per day or higher. Vitamin C is a "fairly" safe vitamin when taken in large amounts, however, taking it in large amounts is really *not* necessary.

Vitamins A, D, C, B6, and niacin may be toxic if taken in large amounts. The recommended safe limits for vitamin A is 10,000 IU or 25 mg per day; for vitamin D, 800 IU per day; for vitamin C, 1,000 mg per day; for B6, 200 mg per day; and for niacin (niacinamide, nicotinic acid, nicotinamide or B3), 500 mg for regular niacin, 250 mg for slow-release niacin, and 1,500 mg for nicotinamide.

Q. Why does my urine turn bright yellow after taking a multivitamin or vitamin B Complex?

A. The excess riboflavin (B2) is the culprit.

Q. How much calcium should be taken daily?

A. For postmenopausal females, studies strongly support the benefit of taking 600 mg of calcium at least twice daily. A multivitamin is unlikely to provide the 1,200-mg necessary to prevent osteoporosis in postmenopausal females, because adding that amount of calcium makes the pill too large. So look for fortified foods or a calcium supplement, to boost what the diet and a multivitamin provide.

Q. Is there a "perfect" multivitamin on the market today?

A. Of course not, however, there are some adequate over-the-counter multivitamins that will suffice for every day supplementation. Not everyone needs every component of a multivitamin. It's also not practical to pinpoint everyone's specific nutrient needs and to come up with an individualized supplement. However, consider your age, your diet and your specific needs and read the labels.

Brand names for general multivitamins that are recommended by most experts include Centrum Advanced Formula, Century Vite, and One-A-Day Maximum. What are the pros and cons of the above three? The pros: the nutrients do not exceed 100% of the daily values. The cons: these could be higher in vitamin C and E.

Theragran M is also recommended, however, it has lower levels of calcium, chromium and magnesium than other multivitamins. Daily One Caps Higher Potency Vitamin and Mineral supplement has more vitamin C and E than most other multivitamins and supplies all of the vitamin A in the less-harmful beta-carotene form. This particular multivitamin, however, is quite expensive and it is lower in calcium and magnesium than other multivitamins.

Dr. Art Ulene of TV fame and fortune has a multivitamin on the market named after himself—Dr. Art Ulene's Nutrition Boost for Men and Women. The pros include antioxidant amounts of vitamin C and E, as well as some "extra" antioxidants such as green tea extract and grapeskin extract. Calcium and magnesium are packaged separately, however, the amounts are still too low to be therapeutic.

Double X Nutrilite (Amway) meets the daily value requirements for magnesium and nearly meets it for calcium. The problem is that calcium is only absorbed 500 mg at a time so the extra calcium may be a waste of money. This multivitamin provides more vitamin C than is necessary, although it's not an excessive amount. An interesting addition to this vitamin is the amount of phytochemicals added to each vitamin. A full two pounds of plant matter is dried and added to each batch. B vitamins are higher than needed in this multivitamin but the amounts are not excessive. This multivitamin also costs megabucks, about $2 bucks a day. Ouch.

Q. Are there specific multivitamins for the over 50 crowd?

A. Yes. Look for a multivitamin that has more B12, is higher in vitamin C and E and calcium, and has *no* or very low iron.

Look at Centrum Silver, even though it is quite low in calcium. It is high in B12 and does not have any iron.

One-A-Day 50 Plus is similar to Centrum Silver but is higher in vitamins C and E. It is also low in calcium.

Dr. Art Ulene's Optimal Vitamin Formula for Men contains plenty of vitamin E, higher calcium than most multivitamins, extra antioxidants, and fish oil for cardioprotection. It does not contain iron.

NOTE: Just remember that most health experts advocate getting nutrients from foods—however that doesn't mean a well-balanced multivitamin/ mineral is a bad idea. It primarily provides insurance against "scurvy" and other nutritional deficiencies. The studies on vitamin B complex, soy, fish oil and others found that the prevention benefits were from food—not a vitamin pill.

MUSHROOMS

Mushrooms. Shiitake and maitake are medicinal mushrooms used to boost the immune system. Mushrooms also come in extracts containing shiitake, maitake, reishi, zhu ling, and others. Check out Fungi Perfecti at 1-800-780-9126 or www.fungi.com for more information on mushrooms.

One mushroom and herb product called PC-SPES has recently garnered a bit of attention in the mainstream journals and news programs. PC-SPES (PC for prostate cancer and SPES for the first four letters of the Latin word for hope) is produced by Botanic lab 1-800-242-5555 or www.pc-spes.com. It contains a combination of nine herbs and mushrooms that are believed to alleviate symptoms of benign prostatic hypertrophy (BPH). This has also been found to be a very promising treatment of advanced prostate cancer that has not responded to conventional hormone therapy (*Journal of Clinical Oncology*, November 1, 2000). PC-SPES contains herbs with phytosterols, quercetin, saponins and polysaccharide compounds, all of which have antitumor effects. PC-SPES costs $10.00-$14.00 per day.

Mango Chutney Dressing
Makes 1-1/4 cups

breakfast · lunch · dinner

    1 cup yogurt – non-fat plain
  1/4 cup mango chutney – prepared
    1 tsp. dijon mustard
  1/2 tsp. vanilla
  1/4 cup apple – cored and chopped

Put all ingredients in a blender or food processor and puree until smooth.

Nutritional info: Serving is 1 Tablespoon: Calories 21; Total fat 0 gr.; Protein 0.8 gr.; Carbohydrates 2 gr.; Fiber 0 gr.; Sodium 12 mg.

is for...
Nutty but Nice

Nuts. *"Sometimes I feel like a nut"*...and you should go ahead and have a handful. What is the relationship of nut consumption and heart disease? Let's look back to the Nurses' Health Study of 86,016 healthy nurses aged 34-59 at study entry in 1980. As of 1990, 1,255 coronary artery events had occurred. After adjusting for the usual risk factors for coronary artery disease (CAD), women who ate more than five ounces of nuts per week had a 35% lower risk of coronary artery disease compared with those who never ate nuts or who consumed less than one ounce per month. The results were the same when the diet was adjusted for all the usual dietary variables—dietary fats, fiber, vegetables, and fruit. The results continued to be the same when the subgroups were stratified by smoking, high cholesterol, alcohol consumption, use of multivitamins including vitamin E supplementation, Body Mass Index and exercise.

Another study of 31,000 individuals found that those who ate nuts more than five times a week lowered their risk of heart disease by more than 50%. Those who ate nuts one to four times per week cut their risk by 27%.

Sounds as if nuts might be the be all and end all for coronary artery disease, eh? Why? Although nuts are high in fat, it just so happens that the fat is mostly monosaturated, which has beneficial effects on cholesterol. However, there's more. Nuts contain arginine, the precursor to nitric oxide, and a potent vasodilator. In addition, nuts contain alpha linolenic acid (an omega-3 fatty acid), which has antiplatelet, antithrombotic, and antiarrhythmic effects. (Hu F, et al. "Frequent nut consumption and risk of coronary artery disease in women: Prospective Cohort Study." *British Medical Journal* 1998 November 18; 317:1332-33. Tunstall-Pedro H. "Nuts to you (...and you, and you): Eating nuts may be beneficial—though it is unclear why." *British Medical Journal* 1998 November 14; 317)

And, nuts not only protect your heart, but a study in the 1999 *Journal of Neurology* found that a diet high in the monosaturated fats contained in nuts can help protect against age-related memory loss and declining cognitive function.

The Nut Museum, 303 Ferry Road, Old Lyme, Connecticut. 860-434-7636; Proprietor: Elizabeth Tashjian. The price of admission for adults—Two dollars and one nut; for kids—one nut.

The museum's most impressive nut is actually the world's largest nut, a 35-pound Coco-De-Mer, grown in the Seychelles Islands in the Indian Ocean. Ms. Tashjian admits that she has a hard time considering the nut as food. "It's difficult, frankly speaking. I start hankering for a pecan and I start cracking it open and I see that it's so beautiful that I can't eat it. I crack open another one hoping that it will break into pieces but that one looks so beautiful too. Before long there is a whole row of nuts and not one has come into my mouth."

Nuts have been food staples for thousands of years. Nut bread was a staple for the great pharaohs, walnuts were used as a remedy for headaches, and newlyweds were pelted with almonds as a fertility blessing. Nuts are chock full of protein, fiber, B vitamins, magnesium, calcium, copper, zinc, selenium, phosphorus and potassium. The fat in nuts is mostly the good guy, monosaturated fat. Almonds and walnuts are also good sources of vitamin E.

A serving size of nuts is one ounce and various nuts have varying nutritional values. The low-fat, low-calorie nut is the chestnut. The high-calorie, high-fat nut is the macadamia nut.

Nutritionist. Need a nutritional advisor in your area? To find one, call the National Center for Nutrition and Dietetics' Consumer Hotline @ 1-800-366-1655.

Keep these on hand to add to salads and grain dishes.

ina's

breakfast • lunch • dinner

Toasted Nuts
Makes 8 servings.

1/2 cup nuts (walnuts, pecans, almonds, cashews, etc.)

Preheat oven to 350 degrees.

Spread the nuts on a baking sheet and toast in the oven for 8-10 minutes. Pay close attention since they burn easily. They should be lightly browned and fragrant.

Cool and store in an airtight container for about 2 weeks.

Nutritional Info: Serving size 1 Tablespoon: Calories 40; Total fat 4 gr.; Protein 1 gr.; Carbohydrates 1 gr.; Fiber 0 gr.; Sodium 1 mg.

---

is for...
Obesity, Onions and Oysters

Obesity and the average American. The average American consumes 64 pounds of fat and oils each year and 65 pounds of sugar. No wonder the average American is *larger* than the average American. In fact, being larger than the average American reduces longevity depending on the actual amount of extra weight carried around. For every seven percent above the ideal weight, reduce the life span by one year. Individuals weighing more than 100 pounds above their ideal weight find themselves fully 50% more likely to die in any given year than their thinner colleagues, friends, and peers. When all of the risks are added together, the risk of dying from obesity in a given year is 1 in 200,000.

FACT: West Virginia. The Centers for Disease Control has proclaimed West Virginia as being the heaviest state in the Union. West Virginia has the greatest percentage of overweight adults—37.8% of the adult population is clinically overweight.

Obesity and cancer. Is fat tissue a risk for cancer? Evidence continues to mount concerning the relationship between obesity and certain types of cancer. In terms of breast cancer, there's no question that gaining weight after menopause raises the risk. Endometrial cancer is also strongly associated with obesity. Eight-five percent of all women who develop cancer of the endometrium are overweight. Obesity also increases the risk for kidney cancer and gastric cancer.

Obesity and depression. In a study from the American Journal of Public Health, obesity was correlated with a 37% higher risk of depression in women and a 37% lower risk of depression in men. Similarly, a 10-unit increase in Body Mass Index (BMI) was associated with a 22% increase in thoughts of suicide and suicide attempts in women, but a 26% and 55% decrease, respectively, in men. Underweight men had a marked increase in depression (25%), thoughts of suicide (81%), and suicide attempts (77%). Once again, which came first? Do extremes in BMI lead to depression or does depression lead to extremes in BMI? The implications are obvious in terms of screening gender for risk factors for depression and suicide. (*Amerian Journalof Public Health* {February}: 90(2): 2000)

Obesity and longevity. In 1997, The Cooper Institute for Aerobics Research in Dallas found that obese people who exercise regularly are less likely to die prematurely than thin people with poor physical fitness.

Obesity and men—the perils of being portly. In a survey of 1,981 men aged 51-88, 24% reported moderate to severe erectile dysfunction (ED). The men with ED were more likely to be older, have hypertension, and weigh more than their study counterparts. Men with waistlines measuring 42 inches were found to be *twice* as likely to suffer from ED compared to men whose girth measured 32 inches. Men who were sedentary were also *twice* as likely to suffer from ED as men who exercised at least 30 minutes per day. Guys, listen up. Get off that couch, pick up those weights, hit the gym runnin' and call your friendly, local nutritionist. For a nutritionist in your neck of the woods, call 1-800-366-1655.

"Let me put it this way. According to my girth, I should be a ninety-foot redwood." —Erma Bombeck

Obesity and viruses. Do viruses cause obesity? The year was 1990. The place was Bombay, India. The scene was a veterinarian discussing a serendipitous observation with a nutritionist. During the discussion, the veterinarian commented that he had made the observation concerning a lethal viral infection in chicken and their tendency to gain a significant amount of weight prior to their demise. Within a 3-week period from the time they acquired the viral infection to the time of death, the chickens gained 60-75% more fat than the chickens that were not infected. In chickens, the virus appeaed to alter metabolism such that, even with the same food and exercise, infected birds gained more weight than uninfected ones.

The nutritionist, Nikhil Dhurander, found the correlation fascinating enough to continue the research and to look for a human corollary. He moved to Madison, Wisconsin to continue his research. The human counterpart to the chicken virus was found to be Adenovirus-36 (AD-36). After six years of research, he reported his findings to the North American Association for the Study of Obesity.

He found that obese patients (15% of 150 patients weighing 250 pounds or greater) had antibodies to the virus compared to the control group who did not have any antibodies and who were lean. Lab animals injected with AD-36 gained enough weight to be classified as clinically obese. A paradoxical characteristic of the virus is that it appears to cause low cholesterol and triglycerides along with obesity. This is good. Obese individuals with AD-36 antibodies also had lower cholesterol and triglycerides than other obese individuals.

Does this mean that antiviral drugs can be used to reduce weight, or even better, to prevent weight gain? Wouldn't that be the answer to all of our obesity problems? The answer is a resounding "no." Researchers state that the large majority of obese Americans gain their weight the "old-fashioned" way, too many calories and too little exercise. *(ADVANCE for Nurse Practitioner's, November 1997)*

"Smoking is responsible for 400,000 deaths per year...obesity for 300,000 deaths per year. Who should our government sue for obesity deaths? " —Anonymous

---

Obesity in America. Only 50% of our children engage in regular physical activity. One of every four boys and girls engages in no exertional activity at all. Contrasted with a decade ago, today's typical child is five pounds fatter. One in five children are obese. Running a mile takes one full minute longer than it did a decade ago. On the parental side, statistics are not much better. According to a recent national study, only 42% of mothers of children grades one through four exercised at all, and only 48% of the fathers. One in four adults are obese, and nearly half of adults are overweight. It is estimated that 12% of all U.S. deaths could have been prevented with even moderate physical activity. Approximately 60% of adults don't get enough physical activity to benefit their health.

"If lack of activity were an infectious disease with these same kinds of numbers and health consequences, it would be a big deal." —James Hill, Nutrition physiologist, University of Colorado Health Sciences Center

---

Obese moms and neural tube defects. Two studies have demonstrated a link between obesity (prepregnant weight) and the risk of neural tube defects. One study noted a two-fold increase among women with a Body Mass Index (BMI) greater than 29 than women with lower BMIs. This finding was independent of other known causes of neural tube defects including folic acid deficiency, type 1 diabetes, use of diet pills, and even previous pregnancy affected by neural tube defects. The second study confirms these findings. Since as many as 10% of women may be obese prior to conception, these findings are important.

Oat bran. Why is it when a label states that two tablespoons of oat bran is good for you that you will automatically assume that three times that much must be even better for you? This was the case with a 75-year-old man who arrived at the emergency room one evening with bloating and severe abdominal pain. The week before during his yearly physical exam his physician had recommended that he increase his intake of fiber and that two tablespoons of oat bran would be the best way to start. The physican also recommended that each tablespoon of oat bran be accompanied by an eight-ounce glass of water. The older man decided that six tablespoons would be much better for his bowels than two. He forgot that water was to accompany the increase in fiber intake and in just under one week he arrived at the emergency room door with the classic signs of intestinal obstruction.

When an older patient arrives at the emergency room with the classic signs of intestinal obstruction, one of the first thoughts of most ER physi-cians is that the obstruction is due to cancer of the colon. So the gentleman was whisked up to the operating room to remove the 'blockage', most likely caused by a malignancy.

Much to the dismay of the surgeon, the 'blockage' was a two-foot long column of oat bran obstructing the sigmoid colon. Upon removal of the oat bran, the bowels were free to move again. Too much oat bran, without the benefit of the water to soften it and keep the stools soft, overwhelmed the ability of the intestines to move, hence the blockage.

Does anyone need to know the moral of this story?

Obstruction due to dried fruit. Abdominal surgery was performed on a older woman with the clinical diagnosis of obstruction. Once again, since the woman was elderly, it was presumed that the obstruction was due to a malignancy blocking the bowel. However, once the surgeon arrived at the designated area, he found a complete undigested apricot blocking the lumen of the intestine. He was perplexed, naturally, and asked the daughter if she might be able to explain the finding. The woman's daughter stated that she had given her mom some dried fruit several days before. Could it be that the dried fruit absorbed the water and expanded into a mass block-ing the bowel?

As an experiment, the surgeon soaked some dried apricots in water for twenty-four hours. Over that period of time the dried apricots absorbed enough water that they enlarged to the size of a fresh whole apricot, about the size of a golf ball. He speculated that the older woman did not chew the dried apricot adequately and most likely swallowed it in its entirety. Hence, the enlargement of the fruit and the obstruction of the bowel.

So, what's the moral of *this* story? Confucius say "One who chew fruit of loom, stay out of operating room."

Olé Olé Olestra! Oh no, Oh no, Olestra. What is olestra? It depletes the body of carotenoids (antioxidant compounds that have been shown to reduce the risk of cancer and coronary artery disease) as well as vitamins A, D, E, and K. But olestra is also Proctor and Gamble's way of saying, you can eat more FAT-FREE potato chips and *not* worry about the calories—WOW! No guilt chips. Fabulous. But is it? Olestra is a calorie-free fat substitute that is licensed under the trade name of *Olean*. Frito-Lay has licensed olestra for its Doritos WOW!, Lay's WOW! and Ruffle's WOW!. Eating chips with olestra does help cut the fat intake, which in turn, does reduce caloric intake. Unfortunately, most people make up for the missing calories by boosting their intake of other high caloric foods and any calorie savings is lost. But, if you eat WOW!s, don't forget to read the small print. Many a WOW! eater has found that the dreaded side effects of olestra include severe abdominal cramping and "anal leakage." Anal leakage is Frito-Lay's way of saying: diarrhea-that-is-practically-impossible-to-reach-the toilet-on-time-with.

Olive oil (extra virgin). The biggest health benefit of olive oil is that nearly three-quarters of its fat content is monosaturated fats, which lowers LDL-cholesterol (the bad guy) while leaving the good cholesterol, HDL, undisturbed. This makes it a perfect "fat" to use to protect the heart.

O
167

Olive oil and colorectal cancer.
Olive oil protects against colorectal cancer by helping to reduce the amount of deoxycholic acid, a bile salt thought to play an active role in colon cancer development. Meat raises the level of deoxycholic acid. (*Journal of Epidemiology and Cancer Health*, October 2000.)

Which oils are best for your health? Oils low in saturated fat but high in monosaturated fat are considered to be the best for health's sake. Below is a quick chart you can use for percentages of saturated fat (the bad fat) and monosaturated fat (if there is a good fat, this would be the one).

Content	Saturated fat	Monosaturated fat
Canola	6%	62%
Grapeseed	7%	79%
Safflower	9%	12%
Sunflower	11%	20%
Peanut	13%	49%
Corn	13%	25%
Olive	14%	77%
Soybean	15%	24%
Vegetable shortening	26%	43%
Butter	54%	30%

(Source: USDA Nutrient Database: www.nal.usda.gov/fnic/cgi-bin;nut_search.pl)

Omega-3 fatty acids. Can you say seafood? "Seafood, seafood and seafood." Ok, ok, ok. Seafood is rich in omega-3 fatty acid. Which seafood? All seafood? Mrs. Paul's fish sticks? Fried Mississippi catfish? No, not exactly. The types of fish that contain the greatest amounts of fatty acids also tend to have high fat contents. When choosing a fish for omega-3 content, choose a fish with the most omega-3 fatty acids for the least amount of fat. The fish containing the most omega-3 fatty acids, more than 1,000 mg per 3 ½ ounce serving includes anchovies, Atlantic halibut, herring, mackerel, salmon (Atlantic chinook, coho, king, pink, sockeye), sardines, shark, trout (rainbow, lake), and tuna (albacore, bluefin). Fish weighing in between 500 and 900 milligrams include Pacific halibut, rockfish, salmon (chum), smelt, squid, striped sea bass, swordfish, turbot, tuna (yellowfin), and whitefish. Walnuts, green leafy vegetables, canola oil, soybean oil, flax oil and ground flaxseeds as well as tofu are also sources of omega-3fatty acids

The two major omega-3 fatty acids are decohexaenoic acid (also known as DHA), and eicosapentaenoic acid (also known as EPA). Well, you have no doubt heard about the omega-3s in the news, so just what the heck are omega-3 fatty acids? Omega-3 fatty acids are polyunsaturated essential fatty acids found primarily in fish and fish oils. The term "essential" means that we "essentially" need them to live. Unfortunately, this is one of those "essential" things that we do not make ourselves, so we have to obtain them from some other source. And, in this case, the source would be the fish we eat, the flaxseed we grind, or the walnuts we use in our Waldorf salad.

Omega-3s first attracted major scientific attention in 1979 when researchers studied native Greenlanders whose diets consisted mainly of cold-water fish. The risk of heart disease in this population was 50% lower than that of adults in the U.S. who were devouring T-bones and Porterhouses and few, if any, cold-water seafood delights. Numerous studies have since confirmed the cardioprotective benefits of omega-3 fatty acids. The mechanism of action appears to involve a positive effect on the lipoprotein profile with an increase in the "good cholesterol" or high-density lipoproteins, as well as a reduction in triglycerides. The other explanation is that omega-3s are converted to a compound similar to prostacyclin, a naturally-occurring vasodilator that also inhibits platelets. In a 1998 study published in the *Journal of the American Medical Association,* men who ate fish as little as once a week reduced the risk of dying suddenly after a heart attack by 52%.

Omega-3s and bipolar disease. In a recent study in the May 1999 *Archives of General Psychiatry*, patients with bipolar disease received either the omega-3 fish oil or olive oil (as placebo) along with their standard medications, including lithium and depakote. After 4 months, 65% of the omega-3 recipients improved, compared to only 19% of the olive oil group.

Omega-3s and cancer prevention. In addition to cardioprotective effects, omega-3 fatty acids may also play a role in preventing certain cancers as well as enhancing traditional cancer therapies. New evidence suggests that omega-3 fatty acids may also slow the rate of metastatic disease. Women whose diets consist mainly of fish, (Asian women for example), exhibit a relatively low incidence of breast cancer. Clinical studies have demonstrated that fish oils inhibit mammary tumor growth in the laboratory, not only preventing the tumor from growing in the first place, but also reducing tumor size in existing breast cancers.

Omega-3s and rheumatoid arthritis. Omega-3 fatty acids inhibit the production of leukotrienes, inflammatory mediators produced in various tissues, including the joints. This has implications for individuals with chronic inflammatory pain syndromes such as rheumatoid arthritis. A study published by the Arthritis Foundation in 1995 suggested that patients with rheumatoid arthritis who took an omega-3 fatty acid supplement along with their regular arthritis medications had improved pain relief.

Researchers from the University of Washington and the Fred Hutchinson Cancer Research Center examined the diets of 324 women who later developed rheumatoid arthritis. The study also followed 1,245 women who remained free of rheumatoid arthritis and served as the control group. The women who ate at least one to two servings of baked or broiled fish each week were 22% less likely to develop arthritis, compared with those who ate fewer servings of fish. Just eating fish with omega-3 fatty acids also reduced the risk of even developing the disease.

Omega-3s and sockeye salmon. Just one serving of sockeye salmon has 27 times the amount of omega-3 fatty acids than a piece of sole. Alaskan natives whose chief form of protein is salmon have less than one-third of the heart attack rate of U.S. caucasians, even though twice as many of the Alaskan natives smoke cigarettes. Omega-3 fatty acids have anti-inflammatory properties, anti-platelet properties, and anti-arrhythmic properties. Broil it, grill it, panfry or poach it. To get the richest flavor from a salmon fillet, begin cooking with the outside up. There is a layer of fat just beneath the skin, and by starting with the skin side up when you grill or broil fillets, the fat will trickle down into the flesh of the fish, adding flavor and moisture.

Onions. Why do raw onions bring a tear to your eye? When you slice an onion, you damage the cell walls, releasing enzymes and sulfur-containing amino acids that trigger a chemical reaction when they come into contact with each other. These volatile sulfur-containing compounds irritate your eyes and stimulate the tear glands. The irritating chemicals just so happen to be water-soluble and the flowing tears help dissolve them. When you cook chopped onions, these unstable compounds break down. Two helpful hints to reduce the tearing that accompanies raw onion cutting: Hold the onion under cold water while cutting it up and/or chill the onion before peeling it.

Onions most likely possess these tearing compounds as a sort of chemical survival system that keeps predators away. It must have worked—onions and other members of the lily family have survived for thousands of years.

Organic foods. Just what is an "organic food"? Americans pay more than $6 billion per year for these foods, so what are you getting when it says "USDA Organic" on the label? Organic foods are supposed to be grown without herbicides, pesticides, synthetic fertilizers, sewage sludge (ick), hormones, artificial additives, chemicals, or any other "unnatural" substance or preservative. However, until recently, many unscrupulous food growers would slap "organic" on the label and consumers had little assurance that this is what they were getting.

Finally the USDA has released a set of standards for labeling organic foods. The new rules will be in full effect by February 2002. The new rules divide organic products into four categories with products that are advertised as "100% organic" at the top of the list. These products must contain only organic ingredients, excluding water and salt. The next category must contain 95% organic ingredients, once again excluding water and salt. Any of the remaining 5% must be non-agricultural products on an approved list, or non-organically produced products that are not available commercially in organic form. The above new categories can proudly display the new USDA organic seal that most likely took 10 years to develop and another 10 for the government officials to agree on.

The remaining two categories are the "also rans." The first food products in this category can carry the label that says they are "made with organic ingredients" as long as they contain at least 70% organic ingredients. And the last category can list specific organic ingredients on the package but cannot have organic on the label if they have less than 70% organic ingredients.

Are organic foods more nutritious and delicious than non-organic foods? No.

Do organic foods cost more than non-organic foods? Yes, by about 50% in your supermarkets and natural food stores. Organic foods are more expensive to grow and harvest. If you choose not to pay the additional 50% for overhead, make sure that you wash your pesticide-grown produce with soap and water. Just dilute your dish soap with water and give them a scrub. Don't bother with those expensive new produce washes, they don't work any better than a little Joy diluted with tap water.

NOTE: Fungus and molds on foods cause health risks and they are more common on organic crops that don't use fungicides to kill them. A mold that grows on corn and peanuts produces the carcinogen, alflatoxin, and can cause an entire crop to be rejected.

For more information see Appendix B..

"Health nuts are going to feel stupid someday, lying in hospitals dying of nothing." —Redd Foxx

---

ORTHOREXIA NERVOSA

Orthorexia nervosa. Do you spend more than three hours per day thinking about healthy food? Do you care more about the virtue of what you eat than the pleasure you receive from eating it? Have you found that as the quality of your diet has increased, the quality of your life has correspondingly diminished? Do you keep getting stricter with yourself? Do you sacrifice experiences you once enjoyed to eat the food you believe is right? Do you feel an increased sense of self-esteem when you are eating healthy food and look down on others who don't? Does your diet socially isolate you? When you are eating the way you are supposed to, do you feel a peaceful sense of self-control? Do you plan your food for tomorrow today? Do you feel guilt or self-loathing when you stray from your diet?

If you have answered "yes" to one or two of these questions you may have a mild case of orthorexia, an obsession with eating healthfully that becomes so strong it leads to progressively rigid dieting that eliminates crucial food groups and nutrients. If you have said "yes" to four or more questions this means that you are in a bit of trouble concerning your unhealthy obsession with food, and if you answer "yes" to all of the questions, you are out of control and definitely need the services of a trained psychiatric professional.

Orthorexia nervosa is an obsession with the quality of food, not the quantity of food, as is the anorexic. Healthy eating becomes a disease in its own right. Individuals lose sight of their obsessive behavior and they believe that by managing their diet they can ward off illness and live happily ever after. Orthorexia is not present at birth. This condition gradually develops over time as the obsession with diet and eating properly occupies a greater part of the day. An orthorexic will lose all pleasure at a dinner party if she eats a piece of cooked broccoli instead of eating broccoli raw. She will berate herself tirelessly if she eats a spoonful of ice cream. Interested in reading more about this horrifying condition? Read *Health Food Junkies: Overcoming the Obsession with Healthful Eating* by Dr. Steven Bratman, Broadway Books.

Oyster alert. If you like oysters, make sure you cook them well before eating them. Raw oysters are a thing of the past, unless you want to play Russian roulette with your health. Even oysters harvested from regularly monitored beds can make you sick if you don't cook them through and through. A 13-state outbreak of food poisoning in 1998 was traced to raw or undercooked oysters from Galveston Bay, Texas. This outbreak followed a summer of record-breaking heat which most likely spawned a population explosion of the bacteria, *Vibrio parahemolyticus*.

Despite monitoring of water quality and bacteria levels at the harvesting sites, more than 400 people in 13 states reported becoming ill with diarrhea, cramping, nausea, headaches, and vomiting within 24 hours of exposure to the infected oysters. So, it would behoove all of you avid oyster eaters to cook them before you eat them, and walk right by the raw oyster bar. If you are cooking your own oysters (or clams) make sure they are cooked to an internal temperature of 140° F. It's rather tough to use a thermometer with oysters, so just make sure that you cook them another 4 to 6 minutes after the shells have opened.

Oysters and the Doctrine of Signatures. Translations from medical texts from 700 B.C. describe an interesting concept called the Doctrine of Signatures. This doctrine is based on the concept that for every part of the human body there is a corresponding part in the world of nature. The ancient physician-priests used this doctrine as the basis for their medical therapies.

"Oysters are supposed to enhance your sexual performance, but they don't work for me. Maybe I put them on too soon." —Gary Shandling

---

For example, if you had jaundice, you might be treated with a mixture based on eviscerated yellow frog. Liverwort plant, with leaves shaped like the liver, would be the correct treatment for diseases of the liver. The ginseng root, resembling a human body, became known as the "whole-body tonic." And, this of course, brings us to the oyster.

The oyster has long been held in high esteem as an aphrodisiac. Oysters were believed to boost libido, elevate testosterone levels, and increase sperm counts. Is there any truth to this claim? A dish of raw oysters somehow doesn't trigger lascivious thoughts in the average American, but if you look a little closer with the Doctrine of Signatures in mind, the oyster resembles a human testicle—in size, in shape, and in color.

Combine the physical appearance of the oyster with the fact that oysters are nature's most concentrated source of zinc. Zinc contributes to the production of the testosterone and sperm. Normal males with zinc deficiency fail to produce enough testicular testosterone resulting in erectile dysfuntion and low sperm count. Eat your oysters!

O

173

"I will not eat oysters. I want my food dead. Not sick, not wounded, dead." —Woody Allen.

Orange and Sesame Dressing
Makes 1 cup

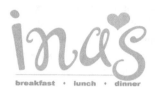

breakfast · lunch · dinner

  1   orange, medium – peeled,
      sectioned and seeded
  1   tsp. honey
  2   Tbsp. balsamic vinegar
  1   Tbsp. lemon juice, fresh
  2   tsp. tahini (sesame paste)
1/2   cup water
  1   tsp. dijon mustard

Place all ingredients in a blender or processor and puree until smooth.

Nutritional Info: Serving is 1 Tablespoon: Calories 11; Total fat 0 gr.; Protein 0 gr.; Carbohydrates 1 gr.; Fiber 0 gr.; Sodium 1 mg.

P is for...
Pizza, Pasta and Prostates

Pizza, pasta, and prostates. Men who eat pizza and pasta with "lotsa" red sauce have a 20% lower risk of prostate cancer. Those who eat at least 10 servings of tomatoes or products made with tomatoes per week, reduce the risk by nearly one-half. Tomato sauce seems to provide more protection than tomato juice. The antioxidant lycopene appears to be the protective substance and tomatoes are the richest dietary source of this particular antioxidant. Cooking the tomato in olive oil improves its absorbability, hence the superiority of tomato sauce over tomato juice.

What about ketchup, you ask? Two tablespoons of ketchup have only 6 mg of lycopene as compared to ½ cup of tomato sauce with 23 mg of lycopene. (*Journal of the National Cancer Institute* 1995; 87:1767)

Packer, Alfred. Alfred Packer's (1842-1907) claim to fame is that in 1873 he led a party of amateur prospectors through the San Juan Mountains during one of the worst snowstorms of the century. He returned alone, saying that his companions abandoned him. Months afterwards, search parties found the bodies of the missing men, most of which had been stripped of their flesh. Packer was tried, found guilty of murder, and sentenced to 40 years of hard labor. As the judge was issuing his sentence he said, "Packer, you depraved Republican son of a bitch, there were only five Democrats in Hinsdale County, and you ate them all!"

Pancreas. It takes 45 minutes from production to final secretion for digestive enzymes from the pancreas to enter the small intestine.

Parkinsonism from dietary sources. The island of Guam and the island of Guadeloupe in the Caribbean have something in common—an unusually high rate of Parkinsonism. It appears as if some of their traditional foods and teas might be the culprit. On the island of Guadeloupe there is an unusually high incidence among the natives who consume a lot of paw paws, custard apples and herbal teas made from leaves, seeds or bark. These contain "actively insecticidal" neurotoxic alkaloids with presumed sedative and aphrodisiac properties. Parkinsonism has also been reported from Guam (known as the "Guam Syndrome") and has been attributed to a "slow toxin" found in their traditional food. A high prevalence of Parkinsonism has also been reported among Afro-Caribbean and Indian immigrants in England, many of whom continue to eat their own ethnic food. (*Lancet* 354:281, 1999)

P
176

Parsley. Eat some parsley after you eat garlic. The chlorophyll in the parsley helps to neutralize the "garlic breath."

"If a parsley farmer is sued, can they garnish his wages?" —George Carlin

Peas, frozen. Use an unopened bag of frozen peas as a substitute for an ice pack. This bag can readily mold itself to the shape of the body part to which it is applied. If the ice pack or bag of peas is applied over an injured part within five minutes, before any swelling takes place, you may reduce the risk of bruising and reduce edema (swelling).

Peanuts. The peanut most likely originated in Peru around 2000 B.C. Spanish explorers and Portuguese explorers distributed the peanut around the world. It most likely reached the U.S. via the slave trade from East Africa but it may have also made its way up from South America through Central America and Mexico. When peanuts were first cultivated in the United States, they were used for livestock feed to fatten pigs, turkeys and chickens. However, after the Civil War, they gained economic importance thanks to one of the most distinguished African Americans of the nineteenth century—George Washington Carver of the Tuskegee Institute.

After the Civil War the South's economy was in a tailspin. The cotton crops were being destroyed by the boll weevil and by over planting. George Washington Carver showed that the neglected peanut, soybean, and sweet potato could produce hundreds of trade goods and replace soil minerals depleted by cotton. Carver spent most of his life studying the various uses of the peanut, and as a result he single-handedly revolutionized the South's post-war economy.

The number one state producing peanuts today is Georgia, followed by Texas, Alabama, and North Carolina. Former President Jimmy Carter is the most famous peanut farmer in this day and age. Jimmy first sold boiled peanuts on the streets of Plains, Georgia when he was knee-high to a grasshopper, only five years old. After the presidency, he moved back to Plains to run the family farm and peanut warehouse. Of course, one of his greatest contributions to mankind is not the peanut. Jimmy Carter is an extraordinary humanitarian and has led humanitarian efforts all over the world on behalf of the poor and indigent populations. In this country, his work for the Habitat for Humanity is without equal.

Peanut butter. Americans consume 700 million pounds of peanut butter per year. A St. Louis physician who wanted to make a high protein diet supplement for his elderly patients first discovered this gummy yummy spread in 1890. In fact, a sandwich-size 3-tablespoon serving of peanut butter contains 13.5 grams of protein—about the amount in 2 eggs or a 12-oz. glass of milk.

Three tablespoons also contains 4 grams of fiber—about as much as a couple of slices of whole wheat bread. The downside: 3 tablespoons of peanut butter equals 300 calories. Ouch. The upside: peanut butter will remove bubble gum from hair.

Q. Why does peanut butter stick to the roof of your mouth?

A. The high concentration of protein gives it an incredible ability to absorb and hold moisture—in other words, it sops up your saliva.

Peanut butter and allergies. BEWARE!

Peanut butter has become one of the most popular "convenience" foods for children. What's better than a peanut butter and jelly sandwich? Delicious, convenient, and inexpensive. So, what's the problem? As peanut butter becomes more and more popular, the risk of peanut allergy increases in direct proportion to its use. Peanut allergy is not only the fastest growing allergy in the U.S., it also causes more life-threatening anaphylactic reactions than all other food allergies combined. Increased consumption is partially responsible, however, the number of peanut-containing products is also on the rise.

You will be quite surprised to know that peanut sources are rather ubiquitous. They are contained in the diaper rash ointment you are using on your newborn. And, of course, all allergists caution that the earlier the exposure to an allergen, the greater the likelihood that you will develop an allergy to it.

How much earlier can you get than a diaper rash ointment? How about breast milk, or other milk formulas? Yes, indeed. The maternal ingestion of peanuts can cross to the infant via breast milk. Peanut oil, by the way, also crosses through breast milk. Fortunately, the grade of peanut oil sold in the United States and Europe contains no detectable proteins and is thus not allergenic. Unfortunately, in other countries peanut oil may contain enough of the protein to cause an allergic reaction.

Other hidden sources include baby massage oil, airplane cabin dust (Southwest Airlines would win the peanuttiest cabin dust award) and skin creams. Peanuts are the base-ingredient for many vitamin D supplements. Small amounts of peanuts may be present in veggie burgers, packaged gravy powder, prepared sauces, and even baked goods. Another recent report warned that even multivitamins have been shown to have peanut oil as one of the ingredients. Some food manufacturers are "de-flavoring" peanuts and disguising them to taste like other nuts. Many of those same companies refuse to guarantee that their products are peanut-free for this very reason. Peanut sensitivity increases the risk of cross-sensitization to other types of nuts and may increase the risk of allergies to milk and eggs.

Families with multiple allergies should be especially aware of the risk of peanuts. Peanuts or food containing peanuts should not be given to children under the age of two. Some experts suggest raising that age to seven in families with allergic histories.

Most fatal anaphylactic reactions to peanuts occur in teenagers, however, the sensitization process usually begins during infancy or early childhood. Children with peanut allergy are most likely to have other related allergic illnesses such as asthma, eczema, and allergic rhinitis.

NOTE: Approximately one in three individuals who has had a near-fatal anaphylactic reaction to peanuts, and who has been rescued with epinephrine, will have a recurrence of anaphylaxis within four hours, and will need a second injection. (*Cutis* 2000 [65]: 285)

If you are allergic to peanuts, carry an epinephrine with you at all times. Even the slightest exposure may trigger anaphylactic shock within minutes of the exposure. One allergic patient used a knife to spread mayonnaise on his sandwich a few days *after* the knife had been used to spread peanut butter on a sandwich. He reacted immediately and developed anaphylactic shock from the exposure to the peanut butter. Families with multiple allergies should be especially cognizant of the risk of peanuts. Peanuts or food containing peanuts should not be given to children under the age of two. Some experts suggest raising that age to seven in families with allergic histories.

Peanuts and genetic engineering. Scientists have identified three genes that code for the allergic proteins found in peanuts. That's the good news. They are using the process of genetic engineering to deactivate these genes and make a non-allergic plant. That's even better news for all of the peanut allergy sufferers in the world.

P
179

PESTICIDES

Pesky pesticides. The benefits of eating fruits and vegetables as a part of your daily diet far outweigh the potential cancer risks from any pesticide residues that are found in the produce you consume. This reassuring data comes from a panel of experts that reviewed over 50 studies and the risks of pesticides. One caveat—high levels of exposure, such as levels that some farm workers are exposed to, *can* pose a substantial risk. The group estimated that all sources of synthetic chemicals, including pesticides, are responsible for 2% of all cancer deaths. Compared to tobacco, which accounts for 30% of cancer deaths, pesticides and friends are a minimal risk.

This is certainly not a carte blanche for eating as many pesticides as you can fit into your diet. It is still important to wash those fruits and vegetables and to reduce exposure to a minimum. (*Cancer*, November 15, 1997)

Apparently there is another way to overdose on those pesky pesticides. In the British journal of gastroenterology, cleverly called *Gut,* a golfer was referred to a GI specialist for unexplained abdominal pains, nausea and lethargy. Upon taking a thorough history, it was revealed that the golfer would lick his golf ball in order to clean it. This procedure resulted in the consumption of pesticide residue. Over time the accumulation of pesticides resulted in his gastrointestinal symptoms of abdominal pains and nausea. His symptoms disappeared when he switched to using a damp cloth to wipe his golf ball. No comment.

Phytochemicals. "Phyto" is the prefix for plant. Phytochemicals are actually toxins in plants used to ward off predators, mostly insects. When animals and humans eat plants, the phytochemicals from the plants induce enzyme systems that may allow us to detoxify foreign proteins including carcinogens

---

There's something a bit absurd about taking phytochemicals in a pill when eating vegetables and fruit that are well-prepared and well-presented is one of life's joys, not one of life's miseries. You can't capture it by just popping pills."
—John D. Potter, Professor of Epidemiology, University of Washington School of Public Health and Community Medicine, Head of Cancer Research at the Fred Hutchinson Cancer Research Center in Seattle, WA.

Pica. Pica is a bizarre eating disorder that has been recognized since the days of Aristotle and Socrates. The term "pica" was first coined, however, by the French physician Ambroise Paré in the sixteenth century. Pica is derived from the Latin word for "magpie," a bird known for its voracious and indiscriminate appetite for edible and nonedible substances.

The actual definition of pica is "the chronic, compulsive eating of nonfoods such as earth, ashes, chalk, and lead-paint chips." The definition may also include a "false or craving appetite" or "deliberate ingestion of a bizarre selection of food." Persons suffering from pica display a persistent and compulsive need to eat non-nutritive substances such as clay, dirt, leaves, cornstarch, laundry starch, baking soda, chalk, buttons, ice, paper, dried paint, plaster, cigarette butts, burnt matches, ashes, sand, soap, toothpaste, oyster shells, or even broken crockery.

Names for subclassifications of pica are comprised of the Greek word for the ingested substance and the suffix from the Greek word "phagein," meaning "to eat." The most common pica as well as the most researched is geophagia, or the eating of earthy substances, especially clay. Other types include the ingestion of ice or ice water (pagophagia); laundry starch (amylophagia); hair (trichophagia); gravel, stones, or pebbles (lithophagia); lead paint (plumbophagia); leaves, grass, or other plants (foliophagia); feces (coprophagia); unusual amounts of lettuce (lectophagia); tomatoes (tomatophagia); peanuts (gooberphagia), and raw potatoes (geomelophagia).

As a rule, the populations most prone to pica are children under the age of six, pregnant women, and persons with mental illness, and the mentally retarded. Pica has also been reported in breast-feeding females and individuals with seizure disorders. It may also run in families. Most likely the familial trait is environmental and not carried as a genetic trait.

As mentioned above, eating earth substances such as clay or dirt is known as geophagia. Some African American females in the Southeastern portion of the United States have been known to practice pica with red clay. Some, who have migrated north, have arranged to have their clay mailed from the South to continue the practice. In addition, southern grocery stores have stocked red clay for human consumption. This form of pica can

HISTORICAL HIGHLIGHT

Vincent van Gogh may have suffered from pica. Van Gogh's unnatural craving involved liqueur called absinthe, which contains the chemical thujone. Thujone, a toxin in the central nervous system, is distilled from plants such as wormwood. Not only did he crave the thujone-laced absinthe, but he was also known to crave substances such as camphor. Camphor contains chemicals known as terpenes, 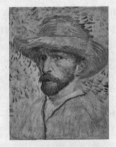 which are also toxic to the central nervous system. He also nibbled on his paints, which contained terpene. Letters from van Gogh to various colleagues substantiated his terpene fetish. One fellow artist had to restrain van Gogh from swilling turpentine one evening.

Both toxins are known to trigger generalized seizures when ingested in large amounts. Van Gogh had at least four documented generalized seizures during the last eighteen months of his life. The accumulation of the toxins in the central nervous system was no doubt responsible for the seizures.

result in an iron deficiency anemia. It is thought that eating clay causes iron deficiency by binding iron in the gut and subsequently inhibiting its absorption. Some clay has been found to decrease iron absorption by 25%. Starch eating has also been associated with iron deficiency.

Pica is a serious eating disorder that can cause gastrointestinal symptoms that require surgical intervention, dental surgery, phosphorus intoxication (from matchhead consumption) or environmental poisoning from lead or mercury that can be contained in the ingested substances. Trichophagia (the ingestion of hair) is found most often in children. It is especially associated with the habit of girls chewing on long hair. Trichophagia can result in substantial amounts of hair being digested and forming "hair balls" in the gastrointestinal tract. These may require surgical removal due to obstruction.

The cause(s) and prevalence of pica are unknown. Estimates in children range from 10-30% in kids from ages 2-6. As a rule kids who engage in pica consume things within the proximity of their grasp. These tend to be relatively harmless items such as cloth, dirt, leaves, sand, rocks and pebbles. Theories abound as to the causes, but include nutritional, physiologic, psychologic and cultural. The most common suspected factors are emotional disturbances and malnutrition resulting from a dietary deficiency.

Nutritional theory suggests that appetite-regulating brain enzymes, altered by an iron, zinc or other mineral deficiency, lead to specific cravings. However, the craved items generally do not supply the lacking minerals.

The physiologic theory notes that eating clay or dirt has been used to relieve nausea, control vomiting, increase salivation, remove toxins, and to alter odor and taste perception.

In terms of psychological theories, pica has been explained as a behavioral response to stress, a habit disorder, or a manifestation of an oral fixation.

And, lastly, pica has been explained as a cultural feature in certain religious rites, folk medicine, and/or magical beliefs. For example, earth taken

FACT: In this day and age, the medical world uses a type of clay as a drug. Kaolinite is the common type of clay used in medicines and the primary ingredient in the commercially marketed antidiarrheal drug known as Kaopectate. Clay is also used medicinally in third world countries where hookworm is a common parasitic infection. This intestinal parasite causes gastric distress that is alleviated with clay. Clay is also used in third world countries to relieve diarrhea, heartburn, and intestinal gas.

from a shrine or holy burial site, is eaten for religious purposes or to swear oaths. (Hunter BT, *Consumer's Research Magazine*, 9/1/97 and the *Cambridge World History of Food*, 2000.)

Pick-a-pie, any pie. Of the three pies—pecan, apple, and pumpkin, which has the most calories per slice? Pecan pie has 500 calories per slice (which is one-eighth of the pie), apple pie has 400 calories per slice and pumpkin pie has 300. How many slices did you have over the holidays? Speaking of holidays, the average weight gain is only about one pound. That's the good news. The bad news is that the pound is usually not lost over the following year. The worst news: Add 20 Christmas and Thanksgiving holidays and you have a 20-pound weight gain. Yikes.

Pickles. You've got to love the name. Pickle. What is a pickle? A pickle is a pickled cucumber. Pickling is a process by which vegetables are steeped in a preservative, usually brine or vinegar. Just about anything can be pickled, including green tomatoes, green beans, cauliflower, carrots, bologna, peppers (as in Peter Piper picked a peck of pickled peppers), pig's feet, beets, onions, eggs, and, the most popular, the cucumber. Pickling has been a popular preservative throughout history, especially before the days of refrigeration and canning. Pickle lovers of yesteryear include Julius Caesar, Napoleon, and Thomas Jefferson. Pickle lovers of today include Barb Bancroft, especially Heinz 57 Processed Dill Pickles.

If you love the sour or dill variety of pickles you will overdose on sodium. One 5-ounce dill pickle has only 24 calories but packs a walloping 1,730 mg of sodium. *Ouch.* The recommended daily allowance of sodium is only 2,400 mg, so you have almost used up your allotment with the one pickle. Enjoy it. So you like the sweet pickles you say? These are definitely lower in salt, but the calories can be as high as 150 in one large sweet pickle. So, pickles, like everything else in life, should be consumed in moderation. Small quantities of thinly sliced pickle chips are fine as an occasional condiment or as a treat right out of the jar.

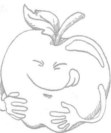

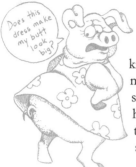

Does this dress make my butt look big?

Pigs and "pigging out." Do pigs pig out? No, only humans pig out. Pigs produce a hormone known as cholecystokinin (CCK), that transmits a message from pork bellies to the pork brains that says, "Stop eating, you pig." Since pigs *listen* to this hormone signal, they do not overeat. Humans have the same signal, however, we typically ignore the message.

Pints and Quarts. We order beer in the U.S. by the bottle or by the glass. In jolly Olde England, ale is ordered in pints or quarts. If a customer was over-served and became a bit unruly, the bartender would holler at them to mind their pints and quarts, or their "P's and Q's."

Piranhas. How fast do they eat? A school of piranhas, which inhabit the freshwater rivers of South America, can chew a 400-pound hog to the bone in less than 10 minutes.

Pistachios. Why are some pistachios dyed red? Pistachios were first mass-marketed in the U.S. in the 1930s during the Great Depression. At that time they were placed in vending machines mixed with the bland cashew nut and the pallid peanut. Some ingenious pistachio manufacturer decided that he would dye them red to make them stand out in the crowd. It worked and pistachios became a hit.

Pomegranate. Humans long ago figured out that certain plants have contraceptive powers. The pomegranate played a central role in both Greek myth and their birth-control efforts. According to the myth, Persephone, the daughter of the fertility goddess Demeter, was told to eat nothing during a visit to the underworld Hades, but she disobeyed and ate the pomegranate. As punishment, the gods sentenced her to spend part of the year in the underworld, and for this reason, Earth experiences the barren season of winter until Persephone returns each spring. The Greeks used the pomegranate as a contraceptive, and studies have found that it contains a plant estrogen that acts like the chemicals found in modern synthetic oral contraceptives.

Popcorn. Constipated? Bad gums? Lousy teeth? Eat one to two quarts of popcorn per day for a safe, inexpensive remedy for all of the above. Americans are the largest per capita consumers of popcorn in the world. Over ten *billion* quarts of popcorn are consumed per year, grossing over one *billion* dollars for the popcorn industry.

Pork. The other white meat. Pork is packed with all of the essential amino acids one needs and it provides plenty of high-quality protein for a nutritious and delicious diet. Pork is a good source of the B vitamins and also provides a bit of heme iron to keep those red blood cells healthy and happy. One broiled lean pork chop has 8 g of fat (2.6 g of saturated fat), 92 mg of cholesterol, and 0.7 mg of iron.

When cooking pork make sure that it has an internal temperature of 170° F. This is hot enough to destroy all of the parasitic roundworms known as *Trichinella spiralis,* the organism that can cause trichinosis. In the U.S. less than 0.5% of the pigs are infected and only 10-100 cases of trichinosis are reported to the CDC each year. Low doses of radiation can also kill this organism, so this may be the safer pork to buy, especially in a high-risk population such as the elderly and immunocompromised.

FACT: Infected hogs are not the only source of *Trichinella spiralis*. If you happen to be visiting the North Pole and you consume polar bear meat, you may also acquire trichinosis from this parasite.

"I had left home (like all Jewish girls) in order to eat pork and take birth control pills. When I first shared an intimate evening with my husband, I was swept away by the passion (so dormant inside myself) of a long and tortured existence. The physical cravings I had tried so hard to deny, finally and ultimately sated...but enough about the pork." —Roseanne Arnold

"BdeBdeBdea..thaaaaaaaaat's all folks." —Porky Pig

Potassium. What are the highest potassium-containing foods? *And don't tell me bananas!* How about potatoes as number one? One medium potato has 755 mg of potassium. One-half of an avocado has 604 mg; ½ cantaloupe has 502 mg; 1 cup of nonfat milk has 408 mg; 2/3 cup of red beans has 340; 1 medium orange has 300 mg and ½ of a banana has 242 mg.

Potatoes (white). The potato is now the fourth most important world food crop, surpassed only by wheat, rice, and maize (corn). Potatoes are inexpensive, nutritious, and a good source of carbohydrates and proteins, while containing minimal amounts of fat. One small potato boiled in its skin provides 16 mg of vitamin C and is therefore an excellent preventive against the vitamin C deficiency known as scurvy. Potatoes are also a great source of B vitamins (thiamine, pyridoxine, folate and niacin) and are a gold mine of potassium, phosphorus and other trace elements. Potatoes provide five grams of fiber if you eat the skin of a large potato. Potatoes are also high in the antioxidants.

Potatoes are members of the nightshade family, Solanaceae, plants that produce neurotoxins (nerve poisons) known as glycoalkaloids. The glycoalkaloid in potatoes is known as solanine, a neurotoxin made in the green parts of the plant, the leaves, the stem, and any green spots on the

The Peruvians of South America, circa 8000 B.C. originally cultivated potatoes. The Spanish explorer Gonzalo Jimenez de Quesada encountered the potato in 1537 in Peru. He has been credited with introducing the potato to the rest of the world. When the potato was first introduced into Europe, it was presumed to be poisonous. However, leading scientists, including Marie Antoinette, tirelessly promoted the potato. In fact, Marie wore potato flowers in her hair in 1785.

Since potatoes were so easy to grow (not a single tool is necessary), they became, as one historian declared, "The difference between having one child and having five." The Irish were the major consumers of the popular tuber and they were consuming eight pounds per person per day by the nineteenth century. Ireland's population doubled but was soon decimated by a potato blight (known as the "late blight") beginning in 1845. Approximately 1 million died, and another 1.25 million immigrated to the United States. The irony of the "late blight" is that it was most likely imported from the United States to England and then Ireland to counter epidemics of other potato blights known as the fungal "dry rot" and the viral "curl" that had plagued previous decades of potato crops. Blight swept Northern Europe, and by 1847, 90% of Ireland's potato crop was diseased. The resulting famine reached its devastating peak in 1847. By 1850, 2 million Irishmen (25% of the population) had either starved to death or had migrated to North America. They sailed to America on "coffin ships" (less room than a coffin), and approximately 200,000 died en route.

In typical American fashion, our country refuses to take responsibility for the deadly fungal infection. A controversial New York State law requires public schools to teach that the British caused the famine.

skin. Solanine interferes with acetylcholinesterase, a neurotransmitter that enables neurons to communicate with one another.

Potatoes exposed to light produce solanine more quickly and in higher amounts than potatoes stored in the dark, but all potatoes produce some solanine all of the time. To prevent greening of the potatoes, store in a dark, cool place that is well ventilated. Solanine persists in the potato even after it is cooked. It is estimated that an adult might have to eat about 3 pounds of potatoes or 2.4 pounds of potato skins at one sitting to experience the first gastrointestinal or neurological signs of solanine poisoning. It is estimated that it would take 1.5 pounds of potatoes or 1.4 pounds of potato skins to cause symptoms in a child. The U.S. government has mandated that potatoes cannot contain more than 200 ppm (parts per million) of solanine per potato. Most potatoes on the grocery shelf contain 100 ppm, however, to be on the safe side, don't buy potatoes with green spots on the skin or potatoes that have sprouts growing out of the eyes.

Don't peel potatoes too far ahead of time, as they will lose some vitamin C to the air and water. In addition, when you cut into a potato the cell walls release polyphenoloxidase, an enzyme that hastens the oxidation of phenols, creating the brownish compounds that darken a fresh-cut potato. To slow down the reaction, soak the peeled sliced fresh potatoes in ice water.

Which potato should be chosen for various potato preparations? Russet potatoes are best for baking and mashing; round red potatoes are the best sautéed; yellow flesh potatoes such as *Yukon Jack* have a dense creamy texture; purple and blue potatoes have a slightly nutty flavor.

Microwaved potatoes or baked in a traditional oven? Microwaving retains slightly more nutrients because of a quicker cooking time than in the traditional oven. Microwaving takes about seven minutes for one medium potato. You'll save nutrients by baking or boiling potatoes in their skins. A potato boiled without its skin loses 8% more potassium, 20% more vitamin C and 5% more B6 than a potato with the skin left on. Bringing the water to a boil before adding the potatoes preserves even more vitamin C.

Potato —other uses. Potatoes have been used to fuel airplanes (potato-based alcohol powered German airplanes in WWII); potato acids are found in detergents; potato starch is used as an adhesive in stamps and as an absorbing agent in disposable diapers. John Dillinger reportedly carved a potato in the shape of a revolver, turned it black with iodine, and used it to escape from jail. Now that's a clever use for a potato.

FACT:
- The ordinary, unruffled potato chip is 55/100 of an inch thick.
- One 15-ounce bag of potato chips = 1 cup of oil.
- A one-ounce bag of chips has about 150 calories.
- One medium movie popcorn (eleven cups) with "butter topping" is the equivalent of eating eight potatoes. It totals 910 calories and 71 grams of fat.
- Each year, McDonald's alone uses 3.2 billion pounds of potatoes.
- Americans eat an average of 2.7 pounds of potatoes per week.

Potato chips: The number one American snack food. A total of 3,468 billion pounds of potatoes are used to make potato chips each year. Another way to put it: 11% of the total United States potato crop becomes potato chips.

Protein. The RDA for protein is 50 grams a day for women and 65 grams a day for men

Protein intake and osteoporosis. Each gram of protein consumed increases calcium excretion by 1 to 1.5 mg. If a woman consumes 65 grams of protein per day, which is the typical amount for the average American woman, she would lose an extra 15 to 23 mg of calcium per day. Over time, this amount of calcium loss adds up and increases the risk for osteoporosis.

Prunes. News Flash from the California Prune Board. As of the fall of 2000, prunes officially changed their name to *dried plums*. The California Prune Board petitioned the Food and Drug administration for a name change and the petition was approved in June. The reason given for the name change: To attract a more youthful market. Thus far there is no evidence that the name change has fooled the youthful market.

Prunes and the bowel. Prunes and prune juice have long been revered by the elderly for their ability to stimulate the bowels. What's in a prune that makes it such an effective laxative? It's certainly not the fiber, even though prunes have a high fiber content. Prune juice has very little, if any, fiber, and it's just as effective as a laxative. So, then, what is it? Apparently it is a derivative of the chemical isatin, which is related to another natural substance, biscodyl, the active ingredient in some over-the-counter laxatives. Biscodyl is a contact laxative that induces the secretion of fluid in the bowel and stimulates peristalsis. Once peristalsis starts, the end result is in the toilet.

Prune profile. Fresh prunes are high in fiber, carbohydrates, vitamin A, folate and vitamin C, and very high in potassium and iron. Dried prunes have everything that fresh prunes have with the unwanted addition of high sodium.

Pumpernickel bread. The word Pumpernickel is derived from the combination of two German words—"pumpern" which means flatulence and "nickel" which is derived from the name of a goblin or devil. Put the two together and you have bread that basically means "devil's fart." Hmmmmm….add a little sauerkraut and corned beef and your cadre of close friends will be severely depleted in no time. One other explana-t i o n is that nickel is an abbreviation of the Christian name Nikolaus (often used in Germany to designate a halfwit). Since pum-pernickel is made with leaven and coarsely crushed pure rye bread, the other name could mean "a coarse bread suitable for a halfwit."

ina's

breakfast • lunch • dinner

"Skinny" French Fried Potatoes
Makes 2 servings

1 tsp. canola or safflower oil
1 baking potato, large - unpeeled and cut into 'French fry' strips

Preheat the oven to 450 degrees.

Using your hand, put about half of the oil in your palm and coat half the potato strips with the oil.

Spread the potatoes on baking sheet in a single layer.

Repeat with the rest of the oil and potatoes and place on baking sheet.

Bake for 15 minutes. Turn them over carefully and continue to bake until evenly browned, about 10 more minutes.

Nutritional info: 1 serving: Calories 93; Total fat 2 gr.; Protein 1 gr.; Carbohydrates 17 gr.; Fiber 2 gr.; Sodium 4 mg.

Q is for...

Quiche Me

Quiche. In Marseille, quiche is a slice of bread spread with anchovies, olive oil, and other selected toppings, and toasted in front of the fire. It is also known as "poor man's cake."

QUERCETIN

Quercetin supplements. In a study reported in the journal *Urology* (54:960, 1999), 500 mg of quercetin twice a day reduced the symptoms of chronic pelvic pain syndrome in 10 of the 15 men taking the supplements. Only 3 of the 13 placebo-taking patients received any relief. What is quercetin? Quercetin is an antioxidant found in small amounts in onions, spices, apples, green tea, potatoes, and red wine.

QUINCE

Quince. Quince is the yellow fruit of a tree native to Asia. In Europe, it is used to make confectionery (candies), liqueurs, and jam.

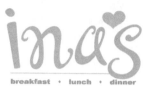

breakfast · lunch · dinner

Pronounced KEEN-WAH, this ancient Andian grain, used as you would a rice or pilaf, has made a come-back in contemporary cook-books and on restaurant menus.

HERBED QUINOA
Makes 6 servings

2-1/2	cups	vegetable stock
1-1/2	cups	quinoa
2	tsp.	butter
3	Tbsp.	Herbs, fresh – chopped
1/4	tsp.	Kosher salt

Bring the stock to a boil in a medium saucepan and add the quinoa and salt. Reduce the heat to low and cover.   Cook for about 15 minutes or until the liquid is absorbed and the grain is tender.

Remove from the heat and add the fresh herbs and butter.

Cover and set aside until ready to serve.

Nutritional Info: One serving: Calories 100; Total fat 2 gr.; Protein 3 gr.; Carbohydrates 19 gr.; Fiber 2 gr.; Sodium 43 mg.

is for...
Red-Dye and
Rum

Red dye number 3. Is it safe to eat foods colored with red dye number 3? Foods such as red M & M's, red cough drops, red pistachios and maraschino cherries? "Yes" is the simple, concise answer. There was a big brouhaha a few years ago about a group of lab rats developing thyroid cancer after consuming amounts of red dye number 3 that would be roughly equivalent to a human eating all the cherries in 2,000 cans of fruit cocktail every day for 70 years. Reason has finally prevailed and our government has declared red dye number 3 to be safe for human consumption.

Refrigeration. Keep the 'fridge between 39° and 40° F, and the freezer between 0°and 5° F. If your settings are 10° colder, the cost of running the refrigerator will be 25% higher than it needs to be. Speaking of the 'fridge...

How about a heart-healthy web site just for women? This web site is sponsored by the American Medical Women's Association and the National Association of Margarine Manufacturer's. Now that's a match, considering margarine's rather poor image as a heart healthy food...oops, I forgot, soft margarines have been vindicated. Anyway, check out www.healthyfridge.org for tips on what to eat, when to eat it, how to eat it, cook it, prepare it, and the latest research on food and women.

Rum. Rum received its name in 1651 when a traveler to Barbados remarked that the islands inhabitants were fond of "Rumbullion alias Kill Devel." Both rumbullion and rumbustion, two early dialect names, may have referred to the violence that the drink was said to cause. Rum became the favorite American alcoholic beverage until the Revolution.

Spicy Rice
Makes 4 servings

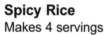

breakfast · lunch · dinner

1	Tbsp. vegetable oil
1/2	tsp. cumin, ground
1/8	tsp. cayenne pepper
3	shallots, large - thinly sliced
1	cup jasmine rice - uncooked
16	oz. chicken broth - canned, low-sodium
1	Tbsp. seasoned rice vinegar
1/4	tsp.Kosher salt

In a medium saucepan, over high heat, heat the oil and stir in the cumin and cayenne. Pull the slices of shallots apart and add to the pan.

Cook, stirring constantly for 2-3 minutes until the shallots soften.

Remove from the pan and set aside.

In the same pan, add the rice and cook, stirring constantly for about 30 seconds. Add the broth, cover and heat to a boil.

Lower the heat to a simmer and cook 15 minutes or until the broth is absorbed.

Turn off the heat and let stand for 5 minutes. Mix in the shallots, vinegar and salt.

Nutritional info: One serving: Calories 240; Total fat 4.7 gr.; Protein 6gr.; Carbohydrates 44 gr.; Fiber 1.1 gr.; Sodium 55 mg.

Sweet n' Salty

Sweet and salty. Why do we love salt and sweets when they are packaged together? Chocolate-covered pretzels are an excellent example of this combination. It would appear as if salt blocks the bitter flavor of foods, allowing the more desirable flavors such as sweetness, to tickle the taste buds. Have you ever noticed that some people salt their grapefruit? This practice enhances the sweetness of the fruit.

SACCHARIN

Saccharin. Saccharin (Sweet'n Low) was discovered in 1879 by a chemist at Johns Hopkins University in Baltimore, Maryland. He noticed a sweet taste on his hands after working with chemicals. (This immediately brings the question to mind, why didn't he wash his hands after working with chemicals? Well, this was 1879 after all.) Since that momentous occasion saccharin has been used to sweeten everything from Tab cola to ice cream and candies. Teddy Roosevelt swore by it and used it in place of sugar because of his diabetes. In fact, he was the champion of saccharin in 1907 when the first attempt was made to ban it due to safety concerns. Saccharin really caught on in the 1960s but as early as 1951 scientists were discussing its carcinogenic potential. In 1977 the Canadian government published a study showing that it caused bladder cancer in male rats. One of the problems with the study was the dose of saccharin used. Those poor rats were exposed to a dose of saccharin that would have caused a bladder tumor in an elephant. Nonetheless, this study set off a maelstrom of controversy and it continues to rage throughout the world of artificial sweeteners.

The diet soft drink industry no longer uses saccharin. Aspartame (Nutrasweet, Equal) has dominated the market for years and is found in over 1,500 products and 90 countries. Aspartame does not cause cancer and doesn't have that bitter aftertaste that saccharin leaves in the mouth. Remember Tab cola? Yuck.

So what's the bottom line here? Studies continue to show that increased rates of bladder cancer are found in individuals who consume foods with saccharin and another artificial sweetener known as cyclamate, as compared to those who don't.

This isn't proof of course, and most researchers believe that saccharin, if it is a carcinogen, is a relatively weak one. So, we still can't let saccharin off the hook totally. In 1997 a panel of experts narrowly voted to recommend saccharin remain on the government's list of "likely" carcinogens.

Historical Highlight

Dr. James Salisbury was a late nineteenth century British physician who practiced and preached preventative medicine, long before it became the vogue thing to do. His major suggestion for disease prevention was to eat well, and that "well" meant to eat well-cooked ground beef three times *per day*. He claimed that this regimen would prevent or cure just about everything that "ailed ya'" at the time, including tuberculosis, heart disease, gout, colitis, asthma, bronchitis, cognitive decline, rheumatism and pernicious anemia. His other "must do" for prevention was to drink a glass of warm water before and after every meal.

S
196

Saliva. Approximately 1 to 1½ liters of saliva are secreted by our salivary glands each day. Most of this saliva is secreted during the day, with very little (about one-tenth) secreted at night. The bacteria that reside in our mouths know this important fact and of course, being the opportunists that they are, they divide more rapidly when we are asleep and our mouths are dry. And just to let you know that they have been busy throughout the night, they leave a nice film covering your teeth as well as a healthy dose of halitosis.

Saliva, one of the body's innate barrier defense mechanisms, has antimicrobial proteins as well as protective secretory IgA antibodies. Those natural protective effects help to explain why HIV is not easily transmitted by kissing or by dental procedures. A new finding provides an additional protective property of saliva—the lack of significant amounts of salt. In fact, saliva has one-seventh the amount of salt as other body fluids. When pathogens are placed in a salt-free environment, the intracellular concentration of salt in the pathogen provides a strong osmotic "pull" from the water-based saliva. Water enters the pathogen causing the cell to literally "blow-up" from water overload.

An important note: Saliva doesn't prevent HIV transmission during oral sex and breast- feeding. The addition of saltier fluids from either of these activities counterbalances saliva's low salinity. (March 1999, *Archives of Internal Medicine*)

Salt and allergic dermatitis. If you've tried everything for your child's eczema and/or allergic dermatitis, try switching their drinking water to bottled water instead of tap water. Tap water contains lots of salt, whereas bottled water does not, and in a few cases it has been shown to be *the* difference, even after trying antihistamines, soothing lotions, and cortisone treatments.

Salt and hypertension. Should everyone reduce salt intake, even if your blood pressure is normal? How much salt should the proverbial "average" American consume in a 24-hour period? The FDA recommends that one should consume *no* more than 100 mg per hour, or cleverly 2,400 mg in a 24-hour day. Since the average American tends *not* to listen to the FDA, what is the average daily intake of salt? It is approximately 4,000 mg per day, a tad above the recommended amount. A recent meta-analysis conducted by researchers receiving financial support from none-other-than the MmmMmm-Good Campbell's Soup Company, reviewed the data collected from 56 clinical trials. Half of the clinical trials involved subjects with hypertension and interestingly enough, the other half of the clinical trials involved patients *without* high blood pressure. Most of the studies had the subjects alternate low-sodium diets with their regular high-sodium diets.

The gist of the research is as follows: Individuals with hypertension received the greatest benefit from low-sodium diets, especially those over the age of 45. Younger individuals with hypertension as well as individuals with normal blood pressures received little, if any, benefit from sodium restriction. (*Journal of the American Medical Association*, May 22/29, 1996).

Salt and osteoporosis. Urinary calcium increases by approximately 23 mg for every teaspoon of salt consumed. An uncompensated calcium loss of 23 mg/day is large enough to dissolve one percent of the skeleton per year. Reducing sodium intake to 1,600 mg/day would lower calcium excretion by one-third. Keep this in mind if osteoporosis is a concern.

Salt and the salt shaker. Just for the record, only 15% of the sodium the average American consumes per year comes from the salt shaker. Another 10% occurs naturally in foods. How then, does the other 75% worm its way into the American diet? Processed foods are the culprits. Especially those easy to pop-in-the-microwave frozen dinners or pizzas, as well as hot dogs, bacon, processed American cheese, canned or dried soups (with

Campbell's MmmMmm Good soups being the absolute worst offenders), salad dressings, canned meats, restaurant and fast foods, just to name a few of the culprits. Just for comparisons' sake:

- Campbell's Vegetarian Vegetable soup – 8 oz. contains 790 mg of sodium *vs* Campbell's Healthy Request Vegetable soup with 500 mg of sodium per 8 oz.
- Celeste Pizza for One, cheese (6.5 ounces) with 1,070 mg of sodium *vs* Weight Watcher's Three Cheese Pizza (6 oz.) with 350 mg sodium.
- Hardee's Chicken Fillet Sandwich at 1,100 mg of sodium *vs* McDonald's McGrilled Chicken Sandwich with 680 mg of sodium.
- Del Monte Whole Kernel Corn, canned (1/2 cup) with 360 mg sodium vs fresh or frozen corn (1/2 cup) with 14 mg of sodium.

Salt surplus. One 325 mg tablet of aspirin contains 70-90 mEq of sodium. This amount must be considered when administered to patients with essential hypertension or sodium-retaining states such as congestive heart failure or renal failure.

One ounce of Cheerios for breakfast provides 333 mg of salt in your daily diet. You might be breathing a sigh relief, thinking, "Whew, I don't eat those unhealthy, salt-laden Cheerios, I'll have the Breakfast of Champions!" Sorry to burst your cereal bowl, but Wheaties are even more salt-saturated, providing 370 mg of salt per ounce. A can of Campbell's Chicken Noodle Soup contains a whopping 980 mg of sodium.

SANDWICH

Sandwich. It is estimated that over 300 million sandwiches are eaten every day in the United States. John Montagu, the Fourth Earl of Sandwich, was born on November 3, 1718, so November 3 has been officially declared as Sandwich Day.

If you want to save a few calories when eating a sandwich, order mustard instead of mayonnaise and save 100 calories. Drop the cheese and save

---

HISTORICAL HIGHLIGHT

John Montagu, the Fourth Earl of Sandwich, invented the sandwich in 1762. Montagu was a gambler and was known for his gambling marathons. On one particular occasion he had been gambling for twenty-four hours and must have been on a winning streak. He didn't want to take the time to eat so he asked his servant to bring the food to the gambling table. He asked that the meat be served between two slices of bread so that he could have one hand free to continue betting. This was a first, and that's how the sandwich was invented.

another 100 calories. Which sandwich do you order most often? As far as healthy eating is concerned, the best bet is a turkey sandwich, no cheese or mayonnaise and placed between two pieces of whole wheat bread.

Sardines. It may come as a shock to many food aficionados, but there is no such fish as a sardine. The term "sardine" is a generic name for a number of small fish such as herring and smelt. The small fish does not become a sardine until it has been canned. During the canning process certain oils, brines, and sauces are added which give the small fish the characteristic sardine flavor. Without these additives, sardines would not be palatable to the average American.

Scromboid fish poisoning. A husband and wife eat grilled mahi-mahi and pasta salad for dinner, washed down with a little white wine and a glass of water. Their canine companion eats the leftover mahi-mahi. Within 45 minutes, the husband and wife vomit. The dog vomits. The husband and wife develop diarrhea, headache, fever, rapid pulse and continue to vomit. The dog does the same. All three members of the family improve after taking benedryl. What's the scoop? Is this a food allergy?

This phenomenon is known as scromboid fish poisoning. Of all varieties of fish, the scromboid species (tuna, bonito, and mackerel) as well as dark meat fish, such as mahi-mahi, are most likely to develop high levels of histamine. When fresh scromboid fish is not continuously iced or refrigerated, bacteria may convert the amino acid histadine, which occurs naturally in the muscle of the fish, to histamine. Since histamine is heat-resistant, cooking the fish generally will not prevent illness.

In the case study described above, the fish was imported from Taiwan through California, and shipped frozen to Albuquerque where it was subsequently thawed and sold from a refrigerated case. Presumably somewhere along the line there was a lack of continuous freezing, allowing the histadine-to-histamine conversion.

Seafood. The average American consumes 15 pounds per year, so what's the best seafood? The seafood that contains omega-3 fatty acids. Think salmon.

Seeds. We're talking about a powerful punch in the world of nutrition. Seeds are filled to the brim with nutrients, including vitamin E, folate, magnesium, copper, manganese and fiber. Seeds are one of the best vegetarian sources of protein, iron and zinc. Does any particular seed stand out? You bet. Sesame seeds are particularly high in calcium, but they also contain copper, manganese, magnesium, iron, thiamine (B1), zinc and B6. Other good choices include ground flaxseed, pumpkin and squash seeds, and sunflower seeds. Remember that seeds are also packed with calories, so you don't want to eat them by the bushel basket. Up to an ounce a day appears to be a practical suggestion. The runner-up in the seed world is the sunflower seed. It has vitamin E, selenium, manganese, copper, pantotheneic acid, folate, B6, niacin and zinc as the bonus ingredients, besides the obvious fiber, protein and fat content. One ounce of sunflower seeds, shelled and dry roasted has 165 calories in it, the same as sesame seeds.

S
200

Selenium in the new millennium. The RDA for selenium is 55 mcg with the UL (upper limit) of 800 mcg daily. Selenium has antioxidant properties and it appears to work in concert with vitamin E in lowering cancer risk, especially of the lung, prostate, and colon. In addition, selenium boosts apoptosis of cancer cells. Apoptosis is the process by which all cells are preprogrammed to self-destruct, a type of cell suicide. Selenium may also activate antitumor substances in cells and/or it may just give the immune system a needed boost to fight cancer.

Selenium is found in high concentrations in foods grown in soils rich in this mineral. Animals grazing on grass grown in selenium-rich soils also have higher concentrations in their meat. Animals may even become toxic on selenium.

HISTORICAL HIGHLIGHT

Marco Polo reportedly was one of the first to report the effects of selenium poisoning during his historical trip to China. After feeding on selenium-rich plants, his horses became so ill the hooves of those most severely affected literally fell off.

AN APPLE A DAY

In areas of the U.S. where the selenium content is low, such as the coastal areas, the rate of prostate cancer is unusually high. Recent research has shown that the incidence of prostate cancer in men who take 200 mcg supplement of selenium is only one-third as high as that of men taking a placebo. In a second study, researchers determined the amount of selenium found in toe-nail clippings and found that men's clippings containing the highest amounts of selenium had the lowest risk of prostate cancer.

Finland recently mandated that selenium be added to all farm fertilizers to reduce the overall risk of cancer. Studies have shown that selenium can also reduce the risk of cancer of the lung, stomach, colon and rectum by as much as 50%. When populations with a low intake of selenium start getting suffi-cient amounts, a reduction in the amount of cancer begins to become evident after three years.

Patients with chronic hepatitis may also want to listen up. Researchers at the National Taiwan University in Taipei studied more than 7,000 chronic hepatitis patients over a 5-year period and found that selenium levels were significantly lower in those who progressed to liver cancer as compared to controls. (*American Journal of Epidemiology*, August 1999)

Selenium and HIV infection. Consider selenium 50-200 mcg per day. A team of Kenyan and U.S. researchers found that women with a selenium deficiency were three times more likely to have HIV shedding in their geni-tal mucosa which may increase their infectivity potential.

"The decline in selenium occurs even in early stages of disease when malnutrition or malabsorption cannot be a problem." (*Lancet* July 2000). What is known about selenium and HIV:

- Less and less selenium is seen as T-cell counts drop.
- People with HIV who also have a selenium deficiency are 20 times more likely to die of HIV-related causes.
- Low levels of selenium are a greater threat to survival than low T-cell counts.
- Selenium deficiency poses more of a risk to survival than low levels of any other nutrient.

Selenium levels. Levels above 10 times the normal amount causes hair thinning and loosening of the toenails and fingernails. (*Lancet* 352:715, 1998.) So watch your hooves if you consume greater than 10 times the normal amount of recommended selenium, or greater than 800 mcg per day. Most of us get plenty of selenium from our diet, so if you are considering a selenium supplement, make sure that your total intake including diet and other supplements such as a multivitamin, does not exceed 800 mcg per day.

The foods containing the highest amounts of selenium are Brazil nuts (4 nuts = 436 mcg), light tuna (3 ½ ounces = 80 mcg), and flounder (3 ½ ounces = 58 mcg) followed by pork, clams, dark turkey meat, white turkey meat, cooked pasta, whole wheat pita bread, Special K cereal, sunflower seeds, granola, Cheerios, English muffins, tofu, whole wheat bread, pinto beans and navy beans. As you can surmise from the list, it's not difficult to get adequate amounts of selenium in our diet in this country.

SERVING SIZE

Serving size. What is the difference between a serving size and a portion size? A serving is a specific, standardized quantity of food based on nutritional need. A portion is whatever is presented to you at a meal. Standard daily servings generally are much smaller than portions served in restaurants or even at home. Here are some easy ways to estimate the recommended serving size:

One half cup of cereal, pasta, potatoes or vegetables is about the size of a small closed fist, a tennis ball, or a billiard ball.

Three ounces of meat, fish, or poultry is about the size of your palm, minus your fingers and thumb; or a deck of cards, cassette tape, or mayo quart jar lid.

One ounce of cheese is a chunk about the size of your thumb, five dice or a ping pong ball.

One teaspoon of peanut butter, butter, mayonnaise or sugar is about the size of your thumb's first joint.

One ounce of snack food is one handful of small foods like nuts, or two handfuls of larger ones like pretzels.

One medium piece of fruit is the size of a baseball or a tight fist.

One medium potato is the size of a computer mouse.

SEX

Sex. Can what you eat influence the sex of your child? Two researchers in the 1970s postulated that certain combinations of electrolytes would influence whether you conceive a boy or a girl. A diet high in salt and potassium, but low in magnesium and calcium would guarantee a boy while the reverse, a diet low in salt and potassium but high in magnesium and calcium would guarantee a girl. Out of 281 pregnancies tested, 83% gave birth to babies of the "right sex." Unfortunately, placebo-controlled studies have *not* confirmed these findings.

SMELL

Smell. Ninety percent of the ability to detect food flavors can be attributed to smell. To check your sense of smell, splurge on 10 different flavors of gourmet jelly beans. With your eyes closed, have another person feed you one flavor at a time and record what flavor you think it is. If you can detect six or seven of the flavors, your sense of smell is probably fine. If you can identify only two or three, see your friendly health practitioner.

Your sense of smell is sharpest in your 30s, 40s and 50s, with a drop-off beginning around age 60. About 50% of people over age 65 suffer some loss of the ability to smell.

FACT: In 1960 it was demonstrated that rats could distinguish schizophrenic sweat from nonschizophrenic sweat. *Trans*-3-methyl-hexenoic acid was found to be the only differing component.

Snacking. The RDA for selenium is 55 mcg with the UL (upper limit) of 800 mcg daily. This results in fewer calories consumed at the subsequent meal and throughout the day. However, if snacking occurs just 30 minutes before the meal, the opposite effect occurs and you will consume more than the normal intake for that meal.

Snacking and kids. One of the explanations for childhood obesity may be sitting right in front of you—easy access to the 'fridge. The study, reported in the April 2002 issue of the *Journal of Pediatrics*, examined snacking habits from 3 surveys conducted in 1977 to 1978, 1989 to1991, and 1994 to 1996. The number of snacks per day increased during the study period from 24% to 32% with the mean daily calorie intake from snacking increasing by 30%. Overall, 77% of children snacked in 1977, and 91% did so in 1996. Hispanic and white children snacked more than black children; a greater proportion of children from higher-income and more highly educated families snacked. Snacks were more energy-dense than meals. Calcium intake declined and iron intake increased significantly in both snacks and meals. Because snacking is so entrenched as a dietary pattern, parents should make a concerted effort to ensure that their children snack on more healthful, less energy-dense foods.

Sniff your patients. Using the old "schnoz" can be a boon to clinical diagnosis if you know the smells you're sniffing around for. The usefulness of the clinician's nose as a part of the physical exam has been around for over 2,000 years. Hippocrates was one of the first proponents of the use of smell for diagnostic purposes.

Some examples of historical uses of odors in diagnosis include the following::

DESCRIPTION OF THE ODOR	DISEASE
Butcher shop	Yellow fever
Freshly baked brown bread	Typhoid
Freshly plucked feathers	Rubella
Putrid	Scurvy
Rotten straw	"Miliary fever" (TB)
Sour or musty bread	Pellagra
Sweetish	Diphtheria

- **Acetone.** The odor of acetone is the hallmark of diabetic ketoacidosis, a complication of type 1 diabetes mellitus. It is described as "fruity," whereas pure acetone is not fruity, but smells like nail polish remover. Theoretically, acetone could be smelled in starvation ketoacidosis (such as those folks on the Dr. Atkins diet), however, these patients are not starving long enough to exhale detectable amounts of acetone.
- **Alcohol.** Because pure ethanol is odorless, it is not possible to smell it on the breath. "Alcohol on the breath" is a term that is misused in all emergency rooms by nurses and physicians alike. What one actually smells is the juniper berry in gin, fusel oil in whiskey, the bouquet of the fermented grape in wine, the hops (a type of flower) in beer, or the acetaldehyde metabolite of alcohol.
- **Ammonia.** Chronic renal failure and liver failure have a characteristic "ammonia" breath, however, the two may be distinguished. In renal failure the kidneys are not capable of excreting dimethylamine and trimethylamine, both of which have a fishy component. In hepatic failure, the breath has a musty, ammonia smell due to mercaptans, dimethylsulfide and dimethyldisulfide.
- **Sewer breath.** Anaerobic bacteria lurking anywhere along the GI tract, from periodontal disease or peritonsillar abscesses to an intestinal obstruction can cause the odor of sewage. Pulmonary infections such as bronchiectasis and pulmonary abscess can also result in this noxious odor.

Soda consumption in the U.S. The amount of soft drinks produced per year in the U.S. is enough to provide a walloping 56.1 gallons per person, which is almost two 12-ounce cans per person daily. Children consume the bulk of the soft drinks in the U.S., chugging at least two to three per day. The amount of soda that we drink per year is twice as much as the amount of beer we drink, more than double the milk or coffee, and six times the amount of fruit juice and tea we drink.

Sorbitol and diarrhea. Halloween diarrhea is a common malady due to the large amounts of sorbitol used as an artificial sweetener in a wide variety of candies. Sorbitol acts as an osmotic diuretic, pulling fluids and electrolytes from the bowels and placing them into the toilet. Diabetics may also consume large amounts of artificial sweetener and may also have diarrhea due to sorbitol. Diabetic diarrhea is usually attributed to autonomic neuropathy, often overlooking sorbitol as a cause. One clue to autonomic neuropathy as the cause—nocturnal (nighttime) diarrhea is usually due to neuropathy and not excess sorbitol.

Sodium bicarb and a full stomach. Sodium bicarbonate (i.e., Arm & Hammer Baking Soda) should not be taken on a full stomach. Case in point: a young gentleman consumed two margaritas, one order of nachos, and a large Mexican combination plate for dinner. Upon arriving home, feeling like a stuffed taco, he gulped ½ teaspoon of baking soda in a glass of water. Within one minute he experienced severe abdominal pain. Emergency surgery revealed a ruptured stomach. It was assumed that once the sodium bicarb hit the hydrochloric acid in the stomach, the combination of the two produced a carbon dioxide gas that was unable to exit the stomach and, BAM!

S
205

Soy and estrogen-dependent cancers. The isoflavones are a mainstay of the Asian diet and their intake is postulated to be a major reason breast and uterine cancer rates are so low in women from Japan, China, and other Eastern countries. The "typical" Japanese woman, living in Japan (versus living in the United States as a Japanese-American), consumes soy products daily, primarily in the form of tofu, produced from soy milk. Numerous studies support the anti-estrogen effects of soy products on the development of estrogen-dependent malignancies in women.

A Brief Digression: This may sound a bit confusing. If soy is a plant-based estrogen, how does it have "anti-estrogen" effects? It is postulated that when bacteria in our intestines metabolize the phytoestrogens, the break-

> **FACT:** John Harvey Kellogg, health guru and cereal king, introduced soybean products in the 1920s as healthful substitutes for milk and meat.

down products exert a weak, but significant estrogenic effect on various tissues in the body. However, these estrogenic effects are different from our own natural estrogens. They may block the effects our own natural estrogens on our tissues. When acting as a partial blocker, the soy isoflavones compete with our own potent estradiol for estrogen receptors on breast and endometrial tissue. In addition, the plant estrogens appear to lower the overall circulating levels of natural estrogen by tricking the hypothalamus and pituitary gland into believing that the body has enough estrogen. This message is relayed to the ovaries and the ovaries slow down the production of natural estrogen.

The first study, reported in the October 4, 1997 *Lancet*, compared 288 women, half of whom had been recently diagnosed with early-stage breast cancer and the other without breast cancer acting as the control group. Researchers compared the levels of various isoflavones in the urine of the both groups and found much higher levels in the control group.

The second study, reported in the August 15, 1997 *American Journal of Epidemiology,* examined the risk factors for endometrial cancer among women from the five main ethnic groups in Hawaii—Japanese, Native Hawaiian, Filipino, Caucasian, and Chinese. Women who ate the most fiber (from cereals, vegetables and fruits), had a 29-46% lower risk of endometrial cancer than women who ate low-fiber diets. The same was true for women who had diets high in soy and legumes. Other phytoestrogen-rich foods, such as whole grains, vegetables, fruits, and seaweeds, also appeared to protect against endometrial cancer.

The isoflavones appear to be more potent than the lignans in terms of protecting the ductal tissue of the breast and the uterine linings. The lignan-containing foods, particularly whole wheat, rye, and flax seeds are also high in fiber and *may* contribute to lowering overall estrogen levels by increasing their elimination from the bowel and reducing intestinal absorption of estrogen.

Should we all rush out and purchase barrels of tofu for immediate consumption? Well, perhaps not barrels, but it may be prudent to gradually add a bit of soy to one's overall healthy diet. The goal should be to work up to 25-45 mg of isoflavones per day taken in food (not supplements). Remember that tofu is 50% fat, so you may want to adjust your fat intake accordingly. The amount of tofu (3.5 ounces) that provides 33.7 mg of phytoestrogens also provides 9 grams of fat, as compared to 3.5 ounces of chicken breast that provides 3.6 grams of fat. On a happier note, tofu has less fat than 3.5 ounces of cheddar cheese (33 grams of fat) and/or extra lean ground beef (16 grams of fat/3.5 ounces). So, how about a tofu burger, hold the cheddar?

Soy and the heart. The isoflavones in soy (genistein, daidzein, and glycitein) are the active ingredients. Consuming soy protein vs. animal protein significantly reduces total cholesterol (9.3%), LDL-cholesterol (12.9%)

and triglycerides (10.5%) while increasing HDL-cholesterol only 2.4%. Genistein acts as an antioxidant, potentially limiting oxidative damage to LDL-cholesterol. Genistein has also been shown to reduce clot formation and to inhibit rapid proliferation of cells following balloon angioplasty.

People with cholesterol levels higher than 240 mg/dL may want to consume 25-50 grams of soy protein daily in place of other protein to reduce their cholesterol levels. The November 14, 2000 issue of *Circulation* has published the first study on the beneficial effects of soy protein consumption to be judged conclusive by the American Heart Association. The study reviewed the latest 38 clinical trials on soy intake and found that 25-50 grams of soy protein per day can safely reduce LDL-cholesterol by up to 8%, reduce triglycerides and increase HDL-cholesterol by 2.4%. The researchers found that soy protein has *no* effect on cholesterol levels under 200 mg/dL.

Soy and osteoporosis. Excessive animal protein increases calcium excretion in the urine. This calcium loss does not occur with consumption of soy protein. Soy protein helps maintain bone density in postmenopausal females. (*Food and Fitness Advisor*, June 2000.)

Soy as a phytoestrogen. Phytoestrogens are actually plant estrogens. Two major classes of phytoestrogens have been defined. Isoflavones found primarily in soy products, and lignans, found primarily in flax seeds, whole grains, and some fruits and vegetables. Tofu has not made the top 10 most favorite foods in the U.S. yet, and for this reason is not a well-known staple of the American diet. Other isoflavones from soy products include roasted soybeans (isoflavone content is 112.5 mg per 3.5 ounces), soy flour (112.4 mg/3.5 ounces), tempeh (62.5 mg/3.5 ounces), textured vegetable protein (38.2 mg/3.5 ounces), and soy noodles (8.5 mg/3.5 ounces.)

New information about estrogen receptors suggests that soy isoflavones activity may be tissue specific, allowing soy isoflavones to have minimal effect in breast tissue. Prior to 1996 it was assumed that there was only one type of estrogen receptor, estrogen receptor alpha (ERa). However, researchers discovered that there were two types of estrogen receptors, ERa and estrogen receptor, beta (ERb). The original ERa occurs at higher levels in tissues in the breast and uterus. The ERbs are located in the cardiovascular system, central nervous system, osteoblasts of the bone, urinary tract, ovaries, testes, kidneys, and colon.

Phytoestrogens, such as soy, have a greater affinity for ERb, allowing them to benefit certain tissues more than others. The discovery of ERb may explain why phytoestrogens such as soy isoflavones appear to provide some of the beneficial effects in the bones, brain and heart, while not causing some of the side effects associated with estrogen excess, such as breast cancer and uterine cancer.

For where to find more information on soy and menopause see Appendix B.

Soy and the thyroid. The FDA has released words of wisdom and words of warning concerning the interaction of soy and thyroid hormones. It appears as if soy can interfere with the production of thyroid hormone. Women with Hashimoto's thyroiditis should minimize their intake of soy products or avoid them altogether, and avoid isoflavone supplements as well.

"Inhabitants of underdeveloped nations and victims of natural disasters are the only people who have been happy to see soybeans." —Fran Leibowitz

---

Space medicine—preparing for the 3-year round-trip to Mars. Space flight *"speeds up aging."* Astronauts experience accelerated bone loss, accelerated muscle loss and a greater chance of DNA mutations that can lead to cancer.

The loss of bone density in space flight equals to approximately 1% per month. The bone loss begins within hours of weightlessness, and is especially pronounced in the weight-bearing bones of the ankles, hips and spine. Using foods with a long shelf life exacerbates the bone loss problem. Shelf-stable foods that would be necessary for such a long flight require large amounts of sodium to remain stable, unlike refrigerated and frozen foods. Unfortunately, more sodium equates to a greater calcium loss from bone. The kidney filters the sodium and it competes with calcium for excretion. Calcium wins the competition and is excreted into the urine and sodium remains in the body. So, until the refrigeration problem is solved, high-sodium shelf-stable foods continue to be the major dietary staple of the astronaut of today.

The lack of the protective ozone layer results in tremendous oxidative damage to the astronaut's DNA, ultimately increasing the risk of loss of growth control and cancer. Providing an antioxidant cocktail containing vitamins C and E, as well as isoflavones from plants may be beneficial.

The risk of colon cancer may be particularly high in the astronaut cohort. Combining the massive oxidative stress with the "fear of flying fiber" provides a fertile soil for DNA mutations and the development of colon cancer. Fiber has been the forbidden food of space shuttles past and present. The prevailing theory was obvious. It would create an overabundance of fecal material with a paucity of disposal space. So the astronauts were given only 0-1 gram of fiber per day, hardly enough to stimulate one centimeter of peristalsis, hence the major complaint of all astronauts was a serious case of constipation.

Adding fish oil to the antioxidant cocktail may help prevent the oxidative damage to cells. Fish oil can potentially prime the cell membrane to signal the rest of the cell that it should prepare to undergo apoptosis, or programmed cell death. This process of apoptosis prevents the precancerous cell from uncontrolled growth and the formation of a malignant tumor.

A second step is necessary to prevent the cancer from developing. The fish oil only *prepares* the cell for apoptosis, it doesn't actually cause the death of the cell. Enter our friend fiber to the tune of approximately 20-25 grams per day. The microflora of the colon "feed off the fiber" and actually form short-chain fatty acids such as butyrate. Butyrate is the "trigger" for the initiation of cell death.

Iron overload is another potential problem on a long space trip. During space travel, astronauts lose approximately 20% of their blood volume. The body compensates by reducing the number of red blood cells, which in turn reduces the amount of intracellular iron. More iron circulates in the blood as "free" iron. Unfortunately this "free" iron may infiltrate organs, resulting in iron overload and tissue damage, similar to the inherited condition known as hemochromatosis.

Muscle atrophy, resulting from the lack of exercise and lack of gravity may be prevented by taking an amino acid supplement. This supplement may also be useful for the elderly who also experience muscle mass atrophy due to disuse and travel medicine sounds exciting, but after realizing all of the potential medical problems, perhaps it's not all it's cracked up to be.

S

209

SPAGHETTI

"Everything you see I owe to spaghetti." —Sophia Loren

Ooh la la. This statement says it all. Perhaps we should all be eating spaghetti on the average of 33 times per day.

SPINACH

Spinach. Each one-cup serving of cooked spinach provides 140% of the day's worth of vitamin A, 30% of a day's worth of folic acid, 15% of a day's iron and vitamin C, and 10% of a day's potassium—and the best part, all of this and more, for only 20 calories. The combination of vitamin C in the spinach is especially nutritive. Vitamin C reduces the loss of folate during the cooking process and it enhances the body's absorption of the iron in spinach. Popeye was on to something, over 70 years ago.

"Spinach poisoning." Spinach contains nitrates that are converted via innate mechanisms in the stomach to nitrites. Nitrites, in turn, react with proteins to form nitrosamines, some of which are known or suspected carcinogens. Before you panic, and eschew spinach for the rest of your born days, this natural chemical reaction presents no known problems for the healthy average American adult. But, when nitrate-rich vegetables (beets, celery, eggplant, radishes, collard and turnip greens, and of course, spinach) are cooked and left to stand at room temperature, bacterial enzyme action (and perhaps some enzymes in the plants) convert the nitrates to nitrites at a much faster rate than normal. These higher-nitrite foods may be hazardous to infants; several cases of "spinach poisoning" have been reported among children who ate cooked spinach that had been left at room temperature for a long period of time.

(c) 2001 King Features Syndicate, Inc. TM Hearst Holdings, Inc.

HISTORICAL HIGHLIGHT

Popeye made his first appearance in the comic strip, *Thimble Theatre*, in 1927. Popeye was not considered to be a major character when he was first introduced. In fact, the original comic strip revolved around his future "goil," Olive Oyl and her family.

Popeye's spinach obsession began in the *Thimble Theatre* comic strip, however, it became an indispensable plot device during his later works as *Popeye the Sailor*. The spinach growers in the U.S. credited Popeye with a 33% increase in spinach consumption, literally saving the spinach industry from ruin.

In 1937, Crystal City, Texas, the spinach capital of the world, erected a statue to commemorate Popeye and his creator, E.C. Segar, and their influence on the spinach-eating habits of the American population.

Stevia (*Stevia rebaudiana*), the "sugar herb." If you are uncomfortable with the artificial sweeteners aspartame and saccharin, Stevia just may be your sweet savior. The FDA allowed Stevia into the country in 1995 with the provision that it must be sold as a dietary supplement, not as an artificial sweetener. The FDA considers it as an untested food additive, although the raw leaves have been used in South America for a few centuries, and processed Stevia has been on the shelves of Japanese grocery stores for over 30 years without adverse effects.

This little green plant native to Paraguay is the sweetest known natural substance. It is 10-15 times as sweet as table sugar, although varying extracts can range from 100-300 times sweeter. If you are going to substitute Stevia in recipes, the conversion rate is one *teaspoon* of Stevia for one cup of sugar. Obviously a mistake here with a one-to-one *cup* ratio would be disastrous for any dessert-loving aficionado.

You can purchase processed Stevia at health-food stores in a concentrated powder or liquid form. You can also grow your own with seeds or plants purchased from your friendly local nursery for about $2-$6 each. Mature leaves can be dried and ground into a green powder to be used in cooking or to sweeten your favorite beverage.

STOMACH

"Anybody who believes that the way to a man's heart is through his stomach flunked geography." —Robert Byrne

STROGANOFF

HISTORICAL HIGHLIGHT

Count Paul Stroganoff was one of the last members of the wealthy Stroganoff family in early nineteenth century Russia. He was famous for his ability to throw lavish dinner parties, many of which featured his now famous signature dish consisting of sautéed beef, onions, mushrooms, sour cream and a few other family secrets. That now famous dish is eponymously known as Beef Stroganoff.

SUGAR

Sugar in all the wrong places. The amount of sugar in one can of soda is 9 teaspoons. Ouch. Nine teaspoons multiplied by 4.5 grams of sugar gives you 40.5 grams of sugar from that one 12-ounce beverage. Non-diet soda is an obvious sugar source as are cookies, ice cream, cakes, pies, soda, and candy bars. The not-so-obvious places will surprise you. Barbeque and steak sauce may have as much as 12-14 grams per teaspoon. Ketchup has 4 grams, however, all brands have varying amounts. A spoonful of jam can give you as much as 14 grams of sugar. Read the labels on cereals. Even some of the so-called all-bran cereals are packed with sugar. Raisin Bran has up to 20 grams of sugar and Wheat Chex has five grams of sugar. Commercial salad dressings have 5 to 7 or more grams and tomato sauces between 11 and 14 grams. Lots of so-called fat-free products are packed with sugar. Jell-O's Fat-free pudding snacks contain 17 grams of sugar. Manufacturers of some fat-free products increase the sugar content to make up for the flavor lost when fats are eliminated, making many of these 'diet, fat-free' snacks higher in calories than the original snack food that contains fat. So, if you are attempting to cut down on your sugar intake, you must, *once again, read the label.*

Sulfites and food allergies. Sulfites (sulfur dioxide, sulfur bisulfite, etc.) are chemicals added to various foods to 1) enhance the flavor (canned tuna, for example), 2) to keep foods from turning brown as they dry (sliced apples, apricots, dried bananas, dried dates, dried figs, dried peaches, dried pineapple, commercially prepared potato salads, dried prunes, and raisins), and 3) to prevent the growth of microorganisms that might turn wine into vinegar. People sensitive to sulfites can have severe allergic reactions, including anaphylactic shock, if they consume these products. In a perfect world, all products containing sulfites should be banned, however, reading the label will provide additional reassurance.

Sulfur and ulcerative colitis. Sulfur in food plays a role in contributing to the abdominal pain and in the frequent hurried trips to the bathroom in patients with ulcerative colitis. One way to help patients with symptomatic ulcerative colitis is to advise them to reduce the amount of dietary sulfur by decreasing the following: whole milk, cheese, ice cream, soy milk, eggs, mayonnaise, red meat, Brussels sprouts, cabbage, broccoli, cauliflower, nuts and wine.

Sweet on sweets. A survey of 400 Americans aged 18 or older shows that that nearly 77% think about dessert between one and eight times per day and 9% have visions of sugarplums dancing in their heads more than eight times per day. In fact, nearly 60% of Americans admit to eating a meal just so they can have dessert and 41% would rather skip the meal and go right for the grand finale. In 1984, the amount of sugar (cane and beet sugar, corn syrup, and glucose) sold in the U.S. was about 125 pounds per person. By 1998, despite the increased use of the artificial sweetener aspartame, the amount of sugar sold per person in the U.S. was 156 pounds. In just 14 years Americans had increased their sweet intake by a remarkable 25%! This averages out to 20 teaspoons per day for the male or female adult and 34 teaspoons per day for the average teenage boy. (*Nutrition Action Newsletter,* September 1999).

According to another survey, 35% of U.S. men and women are not about to abandon all sweets for the sake of the waistline compared to 25% who refuse to give up meat (especially steak) and 14% who draw the line at giving up pizza. Only 7% said that they would consider giving up that good old American staple—the greasy burger.

HISTORICAL HIGHLIGHT

Dentists invented cotton candy and chewing gum, both of which tickle the sweet tooth. Dr. William Morrison, a Nashville dentist in the late 1800s, invented the Fairy Floss candy machine that made sugar-laden cotton candy. About the same time, an Ohio dentist, Dr. William Semple patented the first chewing gum. He anticipated that chewing gum would help clean the teeth… hmmmmmmmmmmmmm. For more fascinating facts on dentistry, visit the National Museum of Dentistry, 31 South Green Street (at Lombard), Baltimore, Maryland. 410-706-8313.

Many new sweets were developed around the turn of the twentieth century. Until that time sugar was very expensive. When the sugar tariffs were lifted in the 1880s, the price of sugar dropped and more people could afford to buy it and experiment with it.

S
213

Jump Start Smoothie
Makes 1 serving

ina's

breakfast • lunch • dinner

1	banana, medium – peeled and frozen
6	strawberries, large – frozen
1/2	peach – peeled, sliced and frozen
1/2	orange, fresh – peeled (leave the white pith) and seeded
3/4	cup soy milk

In a blender, combine all ingredients and process 1-2 minutes until smooth.

Pour into a tall glass and serve.

(Note: Summer is the perfect time to freeze the fruit in individual freezer bags so you can enjoy this Smoothie all winter long!)

Nutritional Info: One serving: Calories 369; Total fat 5 gr.; Protein 10 gr.; Carbohydrates 76 gr.; Fiber 16 gr.; Sodium 29 mg.

is for...

You Say Tomato, I Say Tomah-to

Tomato. "You say tomato, I say tomah-to." No matter how you say it, you should add tomatoes and tomato-based products to your diet, pronto. Tomatoes are rich in lycopene, the pigment that makes tomatoes red. Lycopene is a carotenoid, a plant-based antioxidant compound that protects against cancer and heart disease. In fact, it is more powerful than beta-carotene, the most well-known antioxidant of the bunch.

Should you eat fresh tomatoes for this protective effect or should you pop open a can of tomato paste? This is one case in which canned and processed tomatoes are better than fresh tomatoes. In fact, canned tomato sauce has five times more lycopene than one large fresh tomato. Lycopene develops as tomatoes ripen on the vine. Tomatoes grown for canning are harvested at a riper stage than those sold fresh off the vine. In fact, yellow, orange, or green tomatoes are not good sources of lycopene.

Processed tomatoes are cooked, which makes it easier for the body to absorb the lycopene. In addition, lycopene is fat soluble, so drizzling a little olive oil on fresh tomatoes will help boost lycopene absorption.

FACT: Did you know that the average tomato travels 1,300 miles from farm to salad bowl? (*Environmental Nutrition,* April 2001)

TAB. Can either stand for TAB cola (produced as a diet cola by the Coca-Cola bottling company) or in medicine can stand for Triple Antibiotics—

bacitracin, neomycin, and polymixin. For somewhat obvious reasons the two should not be mixed up. Wounds are irrigated with the antibiotic mix, *not* the diet cola!

Take Control is a cholesterol-lowering margarine substitute containing a stanol ester derived from soybeans. The fatty base is canola and soybean oil. Like Benecol, Take Control blocks the channels in the intestine through which dietary cholesterol passes back into the bloodstream. If cholesterol can't go back into the bloodstream it has only one way to go—into the toilet. Take Control tastes and feels just like regular margarine, however, it cannot be used in cooking since it loses its cholesterol-lowering activity when heated. This is also not considered to be a "weight-loss" product since it contains as much fat as the usual "dose" of margarine. It works best for borderline high cholesterol (in the range of 200-240 mg), and it is not intended to replace cholesterol-lowering drugs. Both Take Control and Benecol work best if the diet contains lots of cholesterol and neither product is effective if you are already on a low animal fat diet.

Tapeworms. Tapeworms derive their name from the fact that the adult worm is long and ribbonlike. The baby worm you accidentally ingest, once it attaches to the wall of the small intestine, may grow to be 60 feet long. Tapeworms can be found in raw meat, undercooked pork and fish.

Gefilte fish, a Jewish delicacy, prepared by boiling ground pike, carp, whiting or other fish that has been seasoned and molded into balls, is a well-known purveyor of tapeworms. When gefilte fish is cooked insufficiently, tapeworm larvae can survive and enter the GI tract of the unsuspecting diner.. Even the Jewish maids developed the tapeworm infection while preparing the gefilte fish and taste-testing the partially cooked fish.

Taste. Four tastes have been traditionally described in the world of taste physiology: sweet, sour, bitter, and salty. However, the taste physiologists have just added a fifth taste to the traditional foursome, umami. U-whoey? Yes, umami (pronounced Oo-mommy.) Actually, the American taste physiologists have arrived just a tad late for the discovery of umami. No less than 1,200 years ago, Japanese cooks described a flavor that they called umami. This flavor is so difficult to describe that it doesn't have a true definition. Some say that it has a "savory characteristic"or that it has a "quality of deliciousness." Other terms used are "rich," "well-rounded," "savory," "full-bodied," and "more chickenlike." The compounds that are responsible for umami have been identified, but each compound has little taste or flavor on its own. However, when added to foods, the natural flavors are enhanced, as is the "quality of deliciousness."

One of the compounds responsible for umami is glutamate or glutamic acid, an amino acid ubiquitous in nature. Amino acids can be combined to form proteins, or they function as a single amino acid. When glutamic acid is not bound to other proteins, it gives food the umami taste. The tomato taste is enhanced by glutamic acid, as are certain cheeses and soy sauce.

MSG, monosodium glutamate, the sodium salt of glutamic acid, has been added to Asian cooking for centuries to enhance the flavors. When MSG is added to meat broth, the overall taste is enhanced and the broth is more flavorful and has a meatier taste. In the 1960s, MSG was reported to be responsible for a collection of symptoms known as the "Chinese Restaurant Syndrome." The symptoms included numbness at the back of the neck and a feeling of pressure in the chest and face. Over the years, MSG has been one of the most intensely studied food additives, and subsequent scientific studies failed to link these symptoms with MSG. As a result of these studies, the American Medical Association's Council on Scientific Affairs, the National Academy of Sciences, and the U.S. Food and Drug Administration have designated MSG safe for human consumption.

Taste buds. The lifespan of a taste bud is about 10.5 days. According to the April 2000 issue of *Psychology Today*, the winter depression brought on by lowered amounts of sunlight can also temporarily blunt the taste buds, making sweet and sour flavors less distinguishable—another reason to be depressed by the lack of winter sunlight.

Taste-altering drugs are the most common cause of taste problems. Some examples include: Captopril (Capoten), Ampicillin, Tetracycline, Cisplatin, Methotrexate, amitriptyline (Elavil), fluoxetine (Prozac), imipramine (Tofranil), pseudoephedrine, clonidine (Catapres), hydrocortisone, levodopa, propranolol (Inderal), albuterol, cromolyn, nifedipine, statins, cholestyramine, clofibrate, gemfibrozil (Lopid), hydrochlorothiazide, baclofen, dantrolene, nitroglycerin patch.

Taste test. To determine your taste perception, place the following in your mouth, one at a time: sugar for sweet, lemon juice for sour, instant coffee granules for bitter, and salt for salty. If you have trouble detecting any of the four, see your health practitioner.

Tea. The Chinese emperor, Shen Nung in 2737 B.C., first discovered tea. He was boiling water outside when some leaves from a nearby bush, the *Camellia sinensis* plant, fell into the kettle. As he was frantically attempting to retrieve the leaves from the boiling water he started smelling a sweet aroma wafting up from the kettle. He tasted it, found it to be delicious, and green tea was invented.

It has been estimated that approximately 2,020,000 metric tons of tea are consumed worldwide each year. This equates to 855 billion cups consumed by everyone around the globe per year. The number one country in the world for producing tea is Kenya, Africa.

The first tea bags were hand-sewn silk bags made by none other than Thomas Sullivan, an American coffee and tea merchant. He would send tea samples in small tin cans to his customers, but this became quite expensive. He decided to save money by putting the tea samples in the silk bags. The customers began ordering their tea packaged in the small bags because they discovered that it was easier to brew their tea in the self-contained packages.

There are many types of tea to choose from today. Green tea, black tea, and oolong all come from the same *Camellia sinensis* plant, but are processed differently. Green tea is made from leaves that are dried soon after harvesting while the leaves are still green. This process gives a delicate flavor to the tea. Black tea is made from leaves that are allowed to ferment after harvesting. The process causes the leaves to oxidize resulting in brownish-black tea leaves and a more intense flavor. Oolong tea is made from leaves that are allowed to ferment for only a short period of time. The taste of oolong tea is somewhere in between green tea and black tea. Black tea is further divided into teas with varying grades of black tea leaves. Souchong, pekoe, and orange pekoe are types of black tea with round leaves, short, round wiry leaves, and wiry leaves, respectively.

The tea plant is a good source of the B vitamin folate. Teas are also high in fluoride, with some tea plants averaging a fluoride concentration of 100 ppm (parts per million). By comparison, fluoridated water has a concentration of 1 ppm. A 5-ounce cup of tea contains an average of 12 mcg of folate, and 0.3-0.5 mg fluoride. Tea also contains a couple of other chemicals called hexanes that inhibit bacterial production of glucans in the mouth. Glucans are a sticky material containing sugar that allows the bacteria to

FACT: It takes 16-24 hours for the bacteria in the mouth to produce the plaque that contributes to gingivitis and periodontal disease. Therefore, brushing after every meal to prevent plaque is an unnecessary expenditure of time and energy. If you brush properly in the a.m. and p.m. and throw in one flossing episode with either, and swish around a mouthful of green tea once a day, plaque problems will be history.

bind to the teeth and cause decay and also contribute to gingivitis and plaque formation. Also, hold a swig of tea (preferably green to reduce staining) in your mouth for 30-60 seconds to reduce plaque formation.

Tea also contains methylxanthine (methyl-zan-theen) stimulants similar to coffee and chocolate. Methylxanthine stimulants include caffeine, theophylline, and theobromine. Coffee has more caffeine and tea has more theophylline. A 5-ounce cup of tea contains 40-60 mg of caffeine compared to a 5-ounce cup of drip-brewed coffee which contains 139 mg of caffeine. Theophylline, by the way, is a drug used to open the airways of patients with asthma and chronic obstructive pulmonary disease. Unfortunately, the relatively low concentrations found in a cup of tea are not therapeutic during an asthma attack.

What happens if you drink too much tea? Too much tea can trigger a thiamine deficiency and a B12 deficiency and can bind calcium and iron into insoluble compounds that your body cannot absorb. The tannins in tea are primarily responsible for these side effects and should be a concern especially in children drinking too much tea. Tea also contains oxalates that can bind calcium and potentially contribute to calcium-oxalate canker sores in those individuals unlucky enough to be predisposed to kidney stone formation. If you can drink your tea with a bit of milk the casein in the milk inactivates the tannins. Also, adding lemon to the tea will inactivate the iron-binding properties of tea.

Teas have been used for medicinal purposes for hundreds of years. Hippocrates recommended a tea made from the bark and leaves of a willow tree for analgesic (pain-killing) purposes. The bark of the willow tree contains salicylic acid, the precursor to acetylsalicylic acid, or aspirin. Tea is a stimulant and mood elevator because of the caffeine it contains. Tea may protect the heart as a result of the B vitamin content. Green tea contains a substance known as epigallocatechin (EGCg) that inhibits an enzyme required for cancer cell growth. In January 1999, Purdue University scientists documented green tea's cancer protective effects. The researchers went so far as to recommend drinking four cups of green tea per day to reduce the overall risk of developing a malignancy.

Tea, herbal. The popular herbal teas are made from the dried leaves or flowers of other plants such as mint or chamomile. The vast majority of the research into the health effects from tea has been done on the traditional teas derived from the *C. sinensis* plant.

Tofu. Just exactly what is tofu? You hear about it, you talk about it, you may or may not devour it with a passion, but where does it come from? Tofu was first produced more than two thousand years ago. It is essentially a cheese made from the "milk" of soybeans, and, it has traditionally been a staple of the Asian diet for centuries. The consistency of tofu is determined by the amount of water left in the curd after pressing. Firm and extra-firm tofu are similar to the tofu produced in China; silken and soft tofu are similar to those produced in Japan.

Tootsie Roll. In 1896, Leonard Hirschfield, a candy-maker in his twenties with a young daughter named Tootsie, introduced the first paper-wrapped candy, the chewy Tootsie Roll.

Tongues. Pink flamingo tongues were considered to be a delicacy in ancient Rome, and blackbird tongues were popular in the Middle Ages. Today, the ox tongue (roughly 4 ½ pounds worth), the calf's tongue, pig's tongue, and lamb's tongue are used for cooking ragouts, stews, and sauces. The calf's tongue is considered to be superior in quality and quicker to cook. I think not.

Total parenteral nutrition. Total parenteral nutrition (TPN) is a method of feeding patients through the veins (also referred to as intravenous or parenteral). In general, TPN is indicated when the gastrointestinal (GI) tract is not functioning properly or bowel rest is necessary for a prolonged period of time. The procedure will benefit patients with various GI ailments such as inflammatory bowel disease, including Crohn's disease and ulcerative colitis, fistula (abnormal connection between bowel loops), and hypermetabolic states with tissue breakdown. Some surgeons will also use TPN for seven days prior to surgery in order to "build-up" the severely malnourished patient. This preoperative procedure has been shown to significantly decrease the rate of surgical complications in this patient population.

TPN provides the patient's daily fluid and caloric needs. Generally it contains free water as well as dextrose (sugar or glucose), lipids (fats), and amino acids (proteins). Dextrose provides 30%-70% of the patient's total caloric needs. The final glucose concentration in the TPN solution should not exceed 35%. Higher percentages increase the risk for clotting and thrombophlebitis. Lipids contribute approximately 30% of the nonprotein calories and provide the essential fatty acids. Providing protein in the form of amino acids helps to prevent muscle breakdown. Electrolytes are also added and include sodium, potassium, chloride, calcium, magnesium, phosphorus, and acetate. Other supplements include multivitamins, trace metals, selenium, and possibly vitamin K (if the patient has liver dysfunction with a prolonged clotting time). Either cimetidine (Tagamet) or ranitidine (Zantac) is also added to help prevent gastric ulcers from excess gastric acid secretion. Insulin is usually added to the final solution to help regulate blood glucose. Most TPN solutions cause hyperglycemia (a secondary diabetes), so insulin is needed to move the excess sugar from the blood into the cells. And finally, heparin may or may not be added, depending on the physician ordering the solution. Heparin has the potential benefit of preventing clots from forming from the hypertonic solution. (Nguyen HQ, Bergerson, SL, Alexander HR. "Internist's guide to total parenteral nutrition." *Internal Medicine* 2000: 21(4): 37-41.)

Triclosan. Triclosan is a chemical bacterial found in many antibacterial soaps. An antibacterial "ingredient" called *Microban* is a trademarked product that incorporates the chemical triclosan as one of its ingredients. *Microban* can be permanently imbedded into cutting boards and dishtowels to inhibit the growth of bacteria like *E. Coli O157:H7* and *Salmonella*.

Don't let this lull you into a false sense of sterile security. While antibacterial products can help keep bacteria at bay, there is no substitute for proper hand washing and other safe food-handling practices. A major concern is the possibility of bacteria developing resistance to yet another antibacterial product.

Truffles. Truffles, which are considered to be one of the most valuable of the edible fungi, grow underground on plant roots and produce volatile molecules that can only be recognized by dogs, pigs and a few other mammals. Humans don't fit into this category of truffle smellers, and therefore pigs and dogs are used to sniff out the underground delicacies.

Tryptophan. Tryptophan, an amino acid, is the building block for serotonin. Serotonin is the "jack-of-all-trades" neurotransmitter. She ("Sara") helps regulate everything from sleep to mood to food intake to pain tolerance. If serotonin levels are low, people complain of insomnia, depression, food cravings (especially carbohydrates), increased sensitivity to pain, aggressive behavior and poor body temperature regulation.

So, when looking at the list of symptoms produced by low serotonin, it would only make sense that there would be a natural tendency to do everything possible to increase serotonin levels. Serotonin levels are directly related to the amount of tryptophan in the diet as well as the availability of vitamins B6, B12, and folic acid.

Paradoxically eating a protein-rich meal (full of amino acids) *lowers* brain tryptophan levels, while eating a carbohydrate-rich snack *increases* brain tryptophan levels. You would think it would be just the opposite, since tryptophan is an amino acid and a protein-rich meal gives you a bolus of tryptophan.

A protein-rich meal provides many other amino acids as well as tryptophan. The "other" amino acids compete with tryptophan for entry into the brain. Tryptophan gets the short end of the stick, so to speak and loses the competition for entry into the brain. If tryptophan is unable to enter the brain, serotonin levels remain low. When serotonin levels are low, a person will crave carbohydrates.

A carbohydrate-rich meal facilitates the entry of tryptophan into the brain. The carbohydrate load stimulates the release of insulin from the pancreas. Insulin causes the competing amino acids to enter body tissues, leaving tryptophan free to enter the brain without competition. Tryptophan is available as the substrate for serotonin production and serotonin levels increase in the brain. The person feels calm, less irritable, happy, and sleepy.

Sugar also triggers the release of insulin from the pancreas. Insulin lowers the serum levels of most large amino acids and increases blood levels of tryptophan. The tryptophan is able to cross the blood brain barrier and induce a short-term increase in brain serotonin levels. That's why a bag of M & M's gives you a quick burst of "feelin' good."

Tube feedings and *Clostridium difficile* infection. Tube feedings increase the risk for *Clostridium difficile* three-fold. The incidence of diarrhea is highest in patients with the feeding tubes that have the tips placed beyond the pylorus (the sphincter between the stomach and the duodenum.) Feeding tubes placed in the stomach appear to benefit from the acidity of the stomach environment.

Although tube feedings have long been associated with diarrhea, it is no longer safe to automatically assume that all diarrhea is "just due to the tube." Prompt efforts should be made, especially in cases of post-pyloric placement, to reveal any *C. difficile* infection. (Bliss D, et al. "Acquisition of *C. difficile* and *C. difficile*-associated diarrhea in hospitalized patients receiving tube feedings." *Annals of Internal Medicine* 1998 (Dec 15); 129:1072-9)

Turkey. Raw turkey breasts are being used in clinical studies to test the efficacy of surgical gloves. Since turkey breasts have a texture very similar to human skin, researchers are operating on turkey breasts to determine how well the gloves block bacteria during operating techniques such as cutting, suturing, and stapling.

Tomato Salsa

ina's

breakfast • lunch • dinner

- 3   tomatoes, medium – cored, seeded and chopped
- 3   scallions, small – trimmed and coarsely chopped
- 1   jalapeno pepper, medium – cored, seeded and finely chopped
- 1   garlic clove – finely chopped
- 1/2 tsp. kosher salt
- 1/3 cup cilantro, fresh – coarsely chopped

Combine all ingredients except the chopped cilantro in a large bowl. Set aside for 1 hour to let the flavors blend.

Just before serving, stir in the chopped cilantro.

Transfer to a serving dish.

Nutritional info: 1 Tbsp.: Calories 4; Total fat 0 g; Protein 0 gr.; Carbohydrates 1 gr.; Fiber 0 gr.; Sodium 36 mg.; Cholesterol 0 mg.

U is for...

UTI and *E. Coli*

Urinary tract infections (UTI) and cranberry juice. Like blueberries, cranberries can also be used as a urinary antiseptic. Cranberries also contain an as yet to be elucidated compound that inhibits the ability of *E. Coli* to attach to the walls of the bladder. If *E. Coli* cannot attach to the bladder wall it cannot trigger a urinary tract infection.

NOTE: An interesting side effect from the Viagra revolution is a 20% increase in urinary tract infections in women whose partners use Viagra. Similar to the "honeymoon cystitis" seen with increased sexual activity after marriage, these women in their 50s and 60s have also experienced an increase in sexual activity since their partner now has a working organ.

Add an ounce of of Vodka to that cranberry juice and give those HDL's a boost while you're at it. ☺

HISTORICAL HIGHLIGHT

One of the first names for the cranberry was "bounce" berry. This name was derived from the fact that ripe cranberries are known to bounce when tossed onto a hard surface. The name "cranberry" was most likely derived from the blossoms resembling the heads of cranes inhabiting the New England bogs and was shortened from craneberry to cranberry somewhere along the way.

USP (United States Pharmacopoeia). Look for a USP designation on a product label which indicates that a supplement meets five quality standards set by the USP for vitamin, mineral, botanical and herbal supplements: 1) disintegration 2) dissolution 3) potency 4) purity and 5) expiration date. Products that say "Laboratory Tested" or "Quality Assured" *don't* meet the standards. Buyer beware.

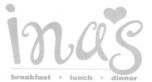
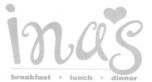

breakfast · lunch · dinner

Spicy Udon Noodles
Makes 4 servings

    12 oz. Udon noodles (or linguine)
     3 Tbsp. rice vinegar
     3 Tbsp. soy sauce
     1 Tbsp. sesame oil, Asian style
     2 tsp. ginger, fresh – peeled and grated
     2 cloves garlic – minced
     1 tsp. sugar
   1/2 tsp. chili oil
     2 green onions – white and green thinly sliced
     1 carrot, medium – peeled and shredded
     1 cucumber, small – peeled, seeded and chopped
   1/4 cup cilantro, fresh – chopped

Bring a large pot of water to the boil and add the noodles. Stir.

Cook according to the package directions.

While the noodles are cooking, mix together all the remaining ingredients.

Drain the noodles and return to the pot. Add the sauce and toss to coat.

Transfer to a serving dish and serve hot or at room temperature.

Nutritional Info: One serving: Calories 351; Total fat 6 gr.; Protein 14 gr.; Carbohydrates 63 gr.; Fiber 4 gr; Sodium 560 mg.

V is for...
Veggies, Vitamins and Viagra

Vegetables. The average American eats only three servings of fruits and vegetables per day—just over half the recommended five servings per day.

Steaming fresh or frozen vegetables in as little water as possible is a great way to retain nutrients. Microwaving works as well as stove-top steaming but be sure to microwave your vegetables in a glass or ceramic container. Microwaving in a plastic container may cause certain chemicals from the plastic to migrate into the vegetables and over the long haul this may be hazardous to your health.

"Vegetables are interesting but lack a sense of purpose when unaccompanied by a good cut of meat." —Fran Leibowitz

---

Valerian *(Valeriana officinalis).* This perennial herb has been used for over 1,000 years as a sleep aid, alias hypnotic/sedative. According to legend, the Pied Piper enticed the rats from the village of Hamelin with valerian, whose volatile oils give it a distinctive, and to most folks, disagreeable smell. In fact, valerian is used to make "stink bombs." Animals love it, hence, the purported use by the Pied Piper.

It may be useful as an over-the-counter herbal remedy for insomnia, mild anxiety, and restlessness. It appears to work by acting as a mild tranquilizer and boosting gamma amino butyric acid (GABA) levels in the brain. It takes a fairly large dose to be effective, typically 50-100 drops of tincture, or a tea prepared from 1 teaspoon of the dried root. This dose may need to be repeated 2-3 times before the desired sedative effect occurs. So it is best to start taking valerian at least one hour before bedtime.

Just a few caveats should be mentioned. Valerian should not be mistaken for Valium. And valerian should not be taken with Valium or any other sedative, hypnotic, or anxiolytic including alcohol. It is not recommended for use with antidepressants either.

Variety is the spice of life. The average American consumes approximately 20 different foods per day.

Vegan. The definition of a vegan is an individual who avoids consumption of any animal foods or dairy products.

Vegans beware. If you are a vegan and avoid any and all animal foods and dairy products, beware of even the most innocuous of food items. Marshmallows and gummy bears have beef and beef byproducts in them. Lipsticks and other cosmetics, cookies, salty snacks, shampoos and ice cream are also rife with meat byproducts. Beef albumin is used in moisturizing creams and the gelatin refined from cattle hide and bones is used in ice cream, gummy bears, and marshmallows. Desiccated liver is used as a nutritional supplement, collagen from the inner layer of the hide is used in cosmetic injections and wound balms, and tallow is used in soaps, creams, and cosmetics.

"Can vegetarians eat animal crackers?" —Anonymous

Vegetarians and wound healing. The diets of some vegetarians may alter the ability to heal normally. Discuss this important fact with any vegetarian planning elective surgery in the future. The vegetarian should consider supplementing the diet for at least one week prior to surgery with the following wound-healing nutrients:
- Albumin contained in proteins
- Glucose contained in carbohydrates

- Essential fatty acids found in walnuts, soybean and canola oil
- Vitamins A, B complex, C, and K
- Minerals including zinc, copper, iron and manganese

Viactiv, the new calcium chew. This is a tasty and convenient way to get the 1,000 to 1,500 mg of bone-building calcium you need daily. Each soft bite-sized candy, at 20 calories and 0.5 grams of fat, supplies 500 mg of calcium, 100 IU of vitamin D, and 50 mcg of vitamin K. The 12-pack of chews costs about $1.50 and they come in two flavors—chocolate and mochachino.

Viagra. Viagra, also jokingly referred to as vitamin V, should not be taken with grapefruit juice. Grapefruit juice increases the bioavailability of Viagra and can result in toxic side effects. Now, it may not seem as if a toxic dose of Viagra would be a bad thing to most gentlemen using this picker-upper. However, blood pressure can fall to dangerous levels especially if other vasodilating drugs are being taken at the same time.

This is actually one of the 3,289 Viagra jokes that has been fired through the internet since Viagra hit the ground running in 1998: Did you hear about the woman who told her husband that she was going to accompany him to the doctor's office when he went for his prescription for Viagra. He turned to her and said, "What are you goin' for?" She replied sweetly, "I'm gonna be gettin' myself a tetanus shot if you're gonna be pullin' out that rusty old thing."

Vinegar. The word vinegar is derived from the French words, *vin* for wine and *aigre* for sour. This was discovered over 10,000 years ago somewhere in France, strictly by accident. Some unsuspecting wine-maker left the wine standing for too long, and made sour wine, or vinegar. The process is slightly more refined today, but essentially requires two steps: 1) yeast changes the natural sugars of the grape to alcohol via the process of fermentation and, 2) bacteria changes the alcohol to an acid via the process of acid fermentation. The wine is then exposed to air for a certain amount of time and voilà, you have vinegar.

Vinegar has been used historically as a medicine and continues to be used today for medicinal purposes. It was prescribed for everything from skin disorders to internal hemorrhaging. Vinegar has been added to water to purify it for drinking. Prior to the days of refrigeration vinegar was used as the preservative in the pickling process.

Vitamin A. The RDA for vitamin A is 5,000 IU (12.5 mg/day). Do not regularly exceed 10,000 IU (25 mg) per day. Retinol and retinoic acid are naturally-occurring compounds with vitamin A activity. This group of compounds is essential for proper vision, growth and cellular differentiation, reproduction, and immune system integrity. Pre-vitamin A carotenoids are beta-carotene, alpha-carotene, and cryptoxanthin. Of the three, beta-carotene is the most important. Carrots and green leafy vegetables provide mega amounts of beta-carotene.

Kids under five are most likely to develop vitamin A deficiency, as are patients with chronic malabsorption. So pump up their intake of carrots and green leafy's.

The earliest symptom of a vitamin A deficiency is night blindness. Once consumed, vitamin A from carrots becomes 11-cis retinol, the essential element in rhodopsin, a protein found in the rods of the retina. Remember, the rods are the cells that help you see in the evening or night. One carrot a day provides more than enough vitamin A to maintain vision in the average American.

WARNING: Vitamin A can cause liver damage and possibly birth defects at daily doses of 10,000 IU or more. The normal human liver contains approximately two year's supply of vitamin A. Because large doses may be teratogenic (causing birth defects), supplementation with vitamin A should be avoided during the first trimester of pregnancy. Liver toxicity occurs in 50% of the patients taking excess vitamin A. The dosage associated with liver damage varies from 15,000 IU per day to 1.4 million IU per day and the duration of exposure from 1 day to 30 years.

HISTORICAL HIGHLIGHT

Beta-carotene is stored in fatty tissue, including the subcutaneous fat just under the skin. During World War II, pilots were fed huge amounts of beta-carotene to improve their night vision. Many pilots developed carotenemia, a yellowish discoloration of the skin, and an indication of beta-carotene excess. Some individuals might mistake this discoloration for jaundice (a yellowing of the skin due to excess bilirubin, the breakdown product of hemoglobin in red blood cells); however, with carotenemia, the sclera (the white membrane covering the eyeballs) are not discolored. Patients with jaundice have yellow sclera, yellow soft palates, and the area under the tongue is also yellow.

Vitamin B1—Thiamine (1.5 mg/day). Do not regularly exceed 50 mg on a daily basis. Foods rich in thiamine include unrefined cereal grains, brewer's yeast, lean pork, legumes, seeds, nuts and organ meats (liver, kidney and heart), as well as foods enriched with B1. Thiamine is a co-factor in carbohydrate metabolism and the need for thiamine is related to carbohydrate intake. Thiamine cannot be stored in the body for any length of time, hence the need to continue to take it in on a regular basis.

Enter the alcoholic. Booze is a well-known source of carbohydrates, however, thiamine has not yet been added to alcoholic beverages. If and when thiamine deficiency occurs, the early symptoms include constipation, decreased appetite, nausea, mental depression, neuropathy and fatigue. As the thiamine deficiency continues, confusion, ataxia (staggering gait), loss of eye coordination and cardiomyopathy (disease of the heart muscle) ensue.

NOTE: If adding thiamine to alcoholic beverages would prevent the acute and chronic problems due to alcohol, one might wonder why this has not been on the agenda of our venerable politicians on Capital Hill. Well, it *has* been on the agenda in years past. In fact, one group that suggested this simple remedy was none other than the government's very own Veteran's Administration Medical Centers. They theorized that adding thiamine to booze would save our Federal Government hundreds of millions of dollars per year in treating veterans with alcohol-related deficiency diseases. Whoa, not so easy, big fella'. The Jim Beams' of Kentucky and Jack Daniels' of Tennessee got wind of the possibility and started pouring in big bucks to the campaign funds of certain powerful congressmen on Capital Hill. The bill didn't even make it out of committee before it was axed. Now you know the "rest of the story." Once again, it doesn't take much to prove the those on "the Hill" rarely, if ever, have two neurons that synapse simultaneously at any given moment.

Vitamin B2—Riboflavin (1.7 mg/day). Do not regularly exceed 200 mg/day. The best dietary sources are animal proteins and green veggies such as broccoli, spinach, turnip greens and asparagus.

Vitamin B3—Niacin (Nicotinic acid 20 mg/day). The recommended safe limit is 500 mg/day (250 mg if it's slow release niacin.) The best dietary sources for B3 are liver, meat, fish, whole grains, poultry, nuts and legumes.

HDL levels increase approximately 20% in patients taking extended-release niacin, also known as Niaspan.

An important note: Flushing is an annoying side effect of niacin—have the patient take a low-dose aspirin 30 minutes prior to taking any formulation of niacin to prevent flushing.

Gradually increase the dose of niacin. Start with 500 mg/day of extended-release niacin each night and increase the dose by 500 mg each month. The usual maintenance dose is 1,500-2,000 mg.

Vitamin B6—Pyridoxine (2 mg/day). The recommended safe limit is 200 mg per day. Pyridoxine is found in fortified cereals, leafy greens, legumes, oranges, chicken, bananas and whole grains. Clinical uses for pyridoxine include:

- The antituberculosis drug, INH, forms complexes with pyridoxine and decreases its availability causing a peripheral neuropathy in some patients. Giving pyridoxine to patients treated with the antituberculosis drug Isoniazid (INH) prevents this side effect.
- Pyridoxine is a safe and effective vitamin for the nausea and vomiting of pregnancy. How is it used? Give pyridoxine (vitamin B6) 25 mg three times a day combined with doxylamine 12.5 mg at bedtime. Doxylamine is a sedating antihistamine and is the main ingredient in Unisom Nighttime Sleep-Aid (but not in any other Unisom formulas). WARNING: Pyridoxine (B6) can cause nerve damage (reversible) at doses of 200 mg or more.
- 2 mg of pyridoxine per day helps to reduce elevated homocysteine levels.

Vitamin B9—Folic acid (200 mcg/day {2 mg} for men; 180 mcg/day {1.8 mg} for women). The recommended safe limit is 1,000 mcg (10 mg) per day. To prevent neural tube defects in women in the "mood or the mode" to get pregnant the dose is 400 mcg or 4 mg per day. The synthetic form is better absorbed than the natural form. Folate is the form found naturally in foods. Lentils, oatmeal, pinto beans, asparagus, and spinach have the highest amount of folate. Folic acid is the form of the vitamin found most often in your body and the form *added* to foods and supplements. Folacin is a collective term for these and other forms of the vitamin. Folic acid has many benefits including:

- **The prevention of neural tube defects.** Neural tube defects occur when the neural tube—which develops the brain and spinal cord—fails to close 18-26 days after conception. If the top of the tube, known as the anterior or ventral opening (neuropore), fails to close, the child does not develop a brain and is usually not carried to full term. If the bottom of the neural tube, posterior neuropore, fails to close, the child has a defect known as a spina bifida (a part of the spinal cord is developed outside the nervous system, usually within a sac on the back of the embryo.)

  The exact mechanism by which folic acid prevents neural tube defects has not been determined, however, folic acid is essential for any tissue that is rapidly dividing. The critical period of neural tube development is only 8 days, and occurs during the first month of pregnancy when most women have absolutely *no* idea that they are pregnant.

Back in 1992, the U.S. Public Health Service recommended that young women who were "in the mood or the mode" to get pregnant should increase their intake of folic acid to help prevent neural tube defects. The folic acid has to be taken prior to pregnancy because the critical period of neural development occurs before most women have any idea that they are pregnant.

By 1996 all grain products were enriched with folate. In the past five years the blood levels of folate have nearly tripled in women of childbearing years. It appears as if this public health measure has been an unqualified success. The number of children born with neural defects has declined by 19% and should continue to fall.(March of Dimes, 2001)

- **The prevention of cardiovascular disease.** As mentioned previously, homocysteine is an amino acid that increases the risk of heart disease. High levels of homocysteine trigger formation of atherosclerotic (fatty) plaques in the coronary, cerebral and femoral arteries. The most important factor affecting homocysteine levels in the general population is a dietary deficiency of vitamin B6 and folic acid. The deficiency of these vitamins causes homocysteine to build up in the bloodstream to rather moderately elevated levels, increasing the risk of cardiovascular disease, stroke, and peripheral vascular disease.

- **The prevention of colon cancer.** It appears as if an ordinary multivitamin containing 400 mcg of folic acid may be enough to offer some protection against colon cancer. The Nurses' Health Study found that nurses who had taken a multivitamin containing folate for at least 15 years had only one-fourth the risk of colon cancer than those who didn't take multivitamins. (*Annals of Internal Medicine* 129: 517, 1998)

There are drugs that inhibit folic acid and may need supplements to overcome the folic acid deficiency. Anticonvulsants such as phenytoin (Dilantin) is a major culprit, however, drugs containing estrogen can also lower folic acid. This estrogen-containing group of drugs includes combined oral contraceptives, and estrogen replacement drugs such as Premarin, Estrace, and Estraderm. Even aspirin has been deemed as one of the "bad guys" when it comes to lowering the folic acid. Seems a bit paradoxical doesn't it? Estrogen replacement and aspirin have always been considered "heart healthy." Lowering folic acid levels results in increased homocysteine levels—not so heart healthy. More studies are needed to determine the clinical implications of these drug-nutrient interactions, however, it wouldn't hurt to take a folic acid supplement if you're on any of these drugs for various and sundry reasons.

Vitamin B12 (cobalamin). The RDA for B12 is 6 mcg per day. Do not exceed 3,000 mcg regularly. No, 3,000 mcg is *not* a typing error. There is a wide margin of safety with B12 doses, unlike vitamins A and niacin. The new guidelines from the National Academy of Sciences recommend that B12 be taken in the synthetic form found in supplements and in food supplemented with B12. The best foods for B12 supplementation are fortified breakfast cereals and dairy products. A bowl of fortified breakfast cereal contains six micrograms of vitamin B12, just the right amount for daily consumption. Contrary to popular belief, B12 from meat, poultry, and fish does not appear to be as effective as supplements. Perhaps some B12 is lost in the cooking process or the way the B12 is bound to the protein in meats may make it less available for absorption (*American Journal of Clinical Nutrition.* 71:514, 2000)

- **B12 absorption and intrinsic factor (pernicious anemia).** When the stomach does not produce intrinsic factor, or when the stomach is too old to want to absorb B12, a deficiency of B12 can be corrected with very large oral doses—1,000 mcg per day. An estimated 1% of the oral dose (100 mcg) crosses the gut mucosa by diffusion and may be sufficient to reverse the deficiency.

- **B12 and anal itching.** One important note: If you do take too much B12 you will have an embarrassing symptom—anal itching. So you might want to cut down on the B12 if this becomes apparent to all of those around you.

- **B12 and depression.** The risk of severe depression was two times higher among disabled women over 65 with vitamin B12 deficiency than among those without the B12 deficiency. The women lived at home, but had at least some difficulty with mobility, exercise, self-care, or other abilities. As a precaution, it is recommended that anyone over 50 years of age should get 25 mcg a day of vitamin B12 from a supplement or a fortified food. (*American Journal of Psychiatry* 2000; 157:715.)

- **B12 and the immune response to pneumococcal vaccine.** Approximately 23% of the older population receiving the pneumococcal vaccine will *not* produce the appropriate antibody response and will thus fail to develop immunity against pneumococcal pneumonia. This may be the result of low levels of vitamin B12. Researchers in New York discovered that none of their patients with low B12 had the capability of producing anti-pneumococcal antibodies.

- **B12 and mental function.** In this study, older individuals with an even marginal B12 deficiency were found to have subtle memory impairment and other mild neurologic cognitive deficits. The author of this study recommends that everyone take 1,000 mcg of vitamin B12 pill daily. B12 is harmless and inexpensive—even when taken in large doses. (*Annals of Internal Medicine* 1996; 124:229, 338.)

Vitamin C. The RDA for vitamin C is 75 mg/day for women and 90 mg/day for men. Smokers should up this amount by 35 mg per day for both genders. The UL for vitamin C is 2,000 mg/day from food and supplements. Any higher than 2,000 mg per day and you might develop a whop-

Dietary treatment for pernicious anemia (low red blood cell production caused by B12 deficiency) was first introduced in the early 1900s. Patients were required to consume at least a half a pound of liver per day as their treatment for this severe, unrelenting (hence, "pernicious") anemia. At the time this replacement treatment with liver was heralded as a lifesaving miracle, even though no one really knew the actual cause of the deficiency.

In 1928, William Castle, a research associate at Boston City Hospital, posed a very simple question: "Why don't normal people need a half of a pound of liver per day to prevent the development of pernicious anemia?" William, (who, by the way, flunked his course in hematology while a medical student at Harvard), knew that the stomachs of patients with pernicious anemia were shriveled and atrophic. He proposed that this atrophic stomach may cause them to lack some very important factor that the stomach could no longer provide.

How did he approach this question? His experimental protocol consisted of two consecutive periods of approximately 10 days, during which daily reticulocyte counts were drawn. (NOTE: A reticulocyte is an immature red blood cell, the precursor to the mature red blood cell known as the erythrocyte. If the bone marrow is making adequate numbers of red blood cells the reticulocyte count should be between 0.5 and 2%.) His study had a sample size of two—himself and one other patient. During the first 10 days the patient received 200 grams of rare hamburger steak daily. His rationale for using hamburger was that it was similar in texture to liver. During this 10-day period the reticulocyte count remained the same.

During the second part of the protocol, Castle consumed 200 grams of hamburger meat. One hour later he inserted a tube through his nose into his stomach (a nasogastric, or NG tube) to collect partially digested contents and gastric juice. He would incubate his gastric contents for several hours until liquefaction of the meat occurred. He then inserted an NG tube into the patient in the study and delivered the solution to the patient. Ick.

The result? The patient demonstrated a rise in the reticulocyte count. In other words, the patient was responding to something that he received from the stomach of Dr. Castle. Castle found that neither the hamburger alone nor the gastric contents, when given alone, would help the patient; they needed to be given in combination in order for the treatment to be effective. He referred to the hamburger meat as the "extrinsic factor" and the substance in the gastric juices as the "intrinsic factor." And now you know the rest of the story. We now know that the "extrinsic factor" is B12, and intrinsic factor continues to be the name of the gastric binding protein that binds the B12 for absorption.

You might be asking yourself, "Why did the one-half pound of liver work by itself as the original treatment for pernicious anemia, but not the hamburger by itself?" Good question, and here's your answer. Liver contains so much B12 that the mass effect of the shear amount of B12 given was enough to ensure sufficient absorption and clinical response despite the loss of binding protein in the atrophic stomach ping case of diarrhea. The recommended intake for health reasons is 200 mg per day not to exceed 2,000 mg per day for prolonged periods. The top 10 foods containing vitamin C are: ½ chile pepper (182 mg), ½ cantaloupe (112 mg), 1 cup orange juice (97 mg), ½ cup sweet red pepper (95 mg), 1 cup grapefruit juice 83 mg), 1 California orange (80 mg), 1 Florida orange (65 mg), 1 cup mixed vegetable juice (67 mg), and 1 cup grape juice (60 mg).

- **Vitamin C as an** antioxidant. The antioxidant dose is 200 mg/day.
- **Vitamin C and the immune system.** Vitamin C minimizes damage to neutrophils (white blood cells) via its antioxidant effects. Vitamin C may also help to mitigate the effects of glucose on cells, thus curbing complications in the patient with diabetes *(Environmental Nutrition,* December 1997)
- **Vitamin C and wound healing.** Vitamin C is necessary for the conversion of the amino acid proline into hydroxyproline, an essential ingredient in collagen. Collagen helps to maintain the integrity of skin, tendons and bones. In an individual with a deficiency of vitamin C, however, replacement with vitamin C may or may not help to speed up the process.

Vitamin D. The recommendation for vitamin D daily is based on age. Individuals up to age 50 should take 200 IUs daily; 51-70 should take 400 IUs daily; and, individuals over 70 should take 600 IUs daily. A multivitamin supplement will usually contain 400 IUs of vitamin D.

Sunlight stimulates the production of vitamin D in the skin, however, we can't rely on Mr. Sun to meet our daily needs. Why? There are many reasons, but probably the most important is our obsession with slathering on sunscreen with SPF's of "2000" every time we venture out into the sunlight. Sunscreens block the ability to convert vitamin D in the skin, while they are protecting the skin from the harmful, cancer-causing rays of the sun. Also, as we age, we become less able to manufacture vitamin D from the sunlight.

People living north of the Mason-Dixon line are also vitamin D-deficient, as are people living in cloudy climates (hello, Seattle and Vancouver), and people living in polluted air (hello, Los Angeles). In Boston, sun exposure does not trigger vitamin D conversion between mid-October and mid-March. In fact, for every ten degrees latitude north, you can add another month at both ends of the season for vitamin D deficiency.

So, you say, I'll just drink more milk fortified with vitamin D. Well, you need a quart a day to get the amount you need and unfortunately that might not be the answer because milk is not a reliable source of vitamin D. Even though vitamin D is added to milk, each carton appears to contain varying amounts of vitamin D. Some cartons are laden with the vitamin and some cartons have minimal amounts.

Ok, then how about a multivitamin, plus sunlight, and a quart of milk? This just might do the trick, but *not* in everyone. In a study reported in the

New England Journal of Medicine (March 19, 1998) 46% of young healthy patients taking multivitamins were deficient in vitamin D, even though the multivitamin contained the recommended daily amount of 400 International Units (IU). Of hospitalized patients, between the ages of 18 and 95, 57% were vitamin D-deficient.

So, what is the bottom line here? How can you tell if you are vitamin-D deficient? The only way to know for sure is to get a blood test for 25-hydroxyvitamin D, an intermediary in the conversion of vitamin D to its active form. Who should have this blood test? Individuals over 50 or if you have risk factors such as living above the Mason-Dixon line, if you are housebound and are not able to get daily or every other day sunlight, and/or if you have chronic liver or kidney disease. If you are over age 50, aim for 800 to 1,000 IU of vitamin D per day. You can combine your sources with multivitamin intake, dietary sources, and a calcium supplement with vitamin D added. Don't go over 2,000 IU per day. Excess vitamin D leads to hyper-calcemia (too much calcium in the blood), which can cause calcium deposits in the kidneys with kidney stone formation and calcium deposits in the arteries and atherosclerosis.

- **Vitamin D and aging.** As we age, our skin becomes 60% less efficient at converting sunlight into vitamin D. Individuals over age 70 should take at least 600 IU with a meal daily. Drinking 6 glasses of milk daily can also provide adequate amounts of vitamin D—each cup of milk provides 100 IU of vitamin D.
- **Vitamin D and Osteoporosis.** It is just as important to have adequate amounts of vitamin D as it is to have adequate amounts of calcium to prevent and to treat established osteoporosis. Vitamin D is essential for the absorption of calcium and for the maintenance of bone mineralization. Some new studies have concluded that as a population, Americans are woefully deficient in this "sunshine vitamin."
- **Vitamin D and Rickets.** This condition is rare in the U.S. however it is occurring more often in breast-fed babies who are not receiving vitamin D supplements or who don't get enough such. African American babies have an increased risk due to decreased vitamin D metabolism secondary to the pigment melanin.

Vitamin E (d-alpha tocopherol or RRR-alpha tocopherol). The recommended daily intake is now 15 mg of alpha-tocopherol for both men and women. However, the recommended "therapeutic dose" for its antioxidant properties is 100-400 IU per day not to exceed 1,000 IU per day. Almonds are the best source of vitamin E, with 11 IU in three tablespoons of almonds. Other dietary sources include walnuts, vegetable oils, liver and leafy green vegetables. But only supplements have the higher amounts that may help reduce the risk of heart disease (100 IU to 400 IU per day) or prostate cancer (50 IU per day). To E or not to E, that is the question.

- **Vitamin E and Alzheimer's disease.** Vitamin E acts as an antioxidant and may prevent damage to neurons and surrounding glial tissue in the brain.
- **Vitamin E and bleeding.** Bleeding complications from vitamin E are quite rare, and are virtually unheard of when the dose is kept at or below 800 IU per day. One note of caution: When other antiplatelet drugs and anticoagulant drugs are used *in addition* to vitamin E, the dose at which bleeding occurs may be less than 800 IU. So, keep in mind drugs such as aspirin, warfarin (Coumadin), ibuprofen (Advil and others), gingko, and garlic.
- **Vitamin E and cancer.** Vitamin E may prevent damage to DNA, the genetic material of the cell, preventing mutations that are likely to result in the loss of control of cell growth.
- **Vitamin E and diabetes.** As an antioxidant vitamin E may help to mitigate the damaging effects of high glucose on cells, thus curbing the complications of diabetes.
- **Vitamin E and the immune system.** vitamin E may protect the cells of the immune system from damage due to the process of oxidation.
- **Vitamin E, heart disease and stroke.** Vitamin E may inhibit the oxidation of the "bad" LDL cholesterol and reduce the build-up of fatty plaques in the coronary arteries. It may also inhibit the ability of platelets to clump (aggregate), reducing the likelihood of a clot.
- **Vitamin E—synthetic or natural?** The recommended daily allowance for vitamin E is 15 mg per day for adults. To get this amount, you need 22 IU of natural vitamin E (also known as d-alphatocopherol) or 33 IU of synthetic vitamin E (also known as dl-alphatocopherol). Why the difference in amounts? Natural vitamin E is more potent than synthetic, so less is needed.

Vitamin K. The current RDA is 80 mcg/day for men and 60 mcg/day for women. Vitamin K plays an essential role in the production of coagulation factors such as prothrombin. Vitamin K is also essential for strong bones. Women should strive for 60 mcg per day and men should shoot for 80 mcg per day. Rich sources of Vitamin K include most dark green leafy greens (kale, lettuce, spinach and Swiss chard), asparagus, broccoli, Brussel sprouts, cabbage cauliflower, and some oils like canola and soybean.

Since Vitamin K plays a major role in the production of prothrombin, should individuals reduce their intake of vitamin K-containing foods if they are on the anticoagulant warfarin (Coumadin). The general answer to that question is no, it's not necessary. However, there may be some situations where your vitamin K intake may increase enough to require an adjustment in Coumadin dosing. What are those situations?

- You don't eat a lot of salads in the winter, but as soon as summer comes around, salads become a daily habit.

- You have started a new diet and have increased your vegetable and salad consumption considerably.
- You are taking *Viactiv*. (Each *Viactiv* chew contains 50 mcg. of vitaminK.)

Vodka. Vodka, meaning "little water," was first distilled in Russia in the sixteenth century from their most abundant grain of the time, rye. Later, in the nineteenth century, potatoes were employed for distillation. Currently maize and wheat are also used for the distillation of vodka in Russia. By 1861 taxes on vodka provided 45% of the revenue of the Russia. Throughout the nineteenth century, more than 70% of the expenditures for the Russian army were paid for by vodka taxes.

Lemon-Dijon Vinaigrette
Makes 2/3 cup

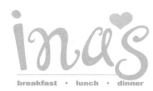

breakfast • lunch • dinner

```
    3   Tbsp. water
    2   Tbsp. lemon juice, fresh
    2   Tbsp. olive oil, extra virgin
1-1/2   Tbsp. red  wine vinegar
    1   Tbsp. dijon mustard
    2   tsp. garlic, minced
    2   tsp. Worcestershire sauce
  1/4   tsp. Kosher salt
Freshly ground pepper to taste
```

Combine all ingredients in a container with a tight sealing lid. Shake well and store in refrigerator.

Nutritional info: Serving is 1 tablespoon: Calories 25; Total fat 2.4 gr.; Protein 0 gr.; Carbohydrates 1 gr.; Fiber 0 gr.; Sodium 93 mg.

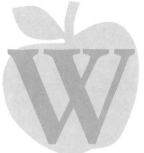

is for…

Wakes, Wine, Wafers and Witchcraft

Wafers, Holy Communion. Often overlooked as a source of wheat gluten, the wafers given out during Holy Communion can be the source of an acute diarrhea attack in individuals with gluten hypersensitivity. Even the wafers classified as "gluten-free" may still contain sufficient gluten to cause diarrhea. Most of the individuals sensitive to wheat gluten are classified as having Celiac disease—an allergy to gluten that results in malabsorption and diarrhea.

Walnuts. Walnuts are full of fat, but eating two ounces of walnuts a day can keep the cardiologist away. Well, that's a slight exaggeration, but walnuts have been shown to reduce cholesterol and LDL-cholesterol. Most of the fat in walnuts is the good guy—polyunsaturated fats. Walnuts are chock full of linolenic acid, which the body converts to heart-healthy omega-3 fatty acids. So, grab a handful of nuts, a small handful (about two ounces) and say cheers to your heart-health!

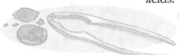

WARFARIN

Warfarin (Coumadin) and nutritional supplements. Many herbs have natural anticoagulant effects that can potentiate the effect of warfarin (Coumadin), and others can counteract its effect. In addition, foods containing vitamin K, a natural antagonist of warfarin, can weaken its effect. Examples include:

- Garlic, dong quai, dan shen, and ginseng can also antagonize the effects of warfarin.
- Gingko biloba is known to contain a potent inhibitor of platelet activation, so that its use with warfarin can cause bleeding.
- Vitamin E has weak antiplatelet effects and is generally not considered to be a problem when taken with warfarin if the dose is less than 800 mg/day.

Green tea has one of the highest contents of vitamin K of any known foodstuff. If taken with warfarin, the patient should limit the intake to only two to four cups of green tea per day. Other vitamin K-rich foods include dark green leafy vegetables such as spinach, collard greens, brussel sprouts and broccoli. Patients can still eat these foods as long as they consume relatively constant amounts since titration of the warfarin dosage takes this consumption into account. Some multivitamin preparations and nutritional supplements such as Ensure and Isocal also contain vitamin K.

Patients should be asked to stop taking any herbs, drugs, or nutritional supplements that potentiate or interfere with the action of warfarin. Those who insist on taking any herb concomitantly with the drug should have an international normalized ratio (INR) measurement within a week of starting to take the herbal product.

WASTING FOOD

Wasting food in America. The average American household wastes up to 15% of the solid food it purchases. The total food wasted in the U.S. would be enough to feed the population of Canada. And, it should come as no surprise, especially to children, that the food most commonly wasted is vegetables.

AN APPLE A DAY

Water. Water is your best choice for replenishing the fluids that are used daily in all bodily functions. Water can even help you lose a little weight. Water is absorbed faster than any other beverage and of course doesn't have any calories. However, don't forget that you get water in foods as well as from drinking a glass of water. Fruits and vegetables contain 80-95% water, milk is 90% water, cooked cereal is 85% water, an egg is 75% water, pasta is 65% water, fish/seafood is 60-85% water, meats are 45-65% water, cheese is 35% water, bread is 35-40% water, nuts are only 2-5% water, and oil is zippo, zero, nada. Foods that are liquid at room temperature can also be counted as fluids. This includes popsicles, sherbet, ice cream and there's always room for Jello. What about booze? No. Booze is a diuretic and causes you to lose more fluid that you take in. How about coffee and soda? If they contain caffeine they cannot be considered as fluid replacement. If they are decaffeinated, they can. Caffeine is also a diuretic and, like booze, increases your fluid needs.

> **FACT:** A person drinks about 16,000 gallons of water in a lifetime.

How do you know how much water to drink? First of all, don't rely on your thirst mechanisms to tell you when to take a swig. If you are thirsty, you have waited too long for that drink. By the time you feel thirsty, you are about two cups low and may already be mildly dehydrated. As we age we also lose our thirst mechanism so we can't even rely on that to tell us when we are mildly dehydrated. So, here are a few ways to keep your water balance where it should be:

1) Hop on a scale, weigh yourself, and divide your weight in half. That number, in ounces, is your recommended daily fluid intake. Adding a slice of lemon or lime is a good way to vary the taste of bottled water. (Cory SerVaas, M.D.)
2) Drink 2/3 ounces of water per pound of body weight per day if you're active and ½ ounce per pound if you are a couch potato. (International Sportsmedicine Institute, West Los Angeles, California.)
3) Another general rule is to drink a quart of water for every 1,000 calories you burn. (*Environmental Nutrition*, May 1998)

Water and bladder cancer in men. Drinking six or more cups of water per day may cut the risk of bladder cancer by 50% compared to men who drink less than one cup a day. It is presumed that potential carcinogens that collect in the urine are more diluted with increased water intake and would therefore result in less contact with the bladder wall. And, obviously, drinking all of that water would have a diuretic effect and wash out carcinogens before they have a chance to damage the DNA of the cells lining the bladder walls.(*N Engl J Med* 340: 1390, 1424, 1999)

Water and rectal cancer. A study from Taiwan found that men who drank the most water (a quart or at least 4 cups in a 24-hour period) had a 92% lower risk of rectal cancer than those who consumed 1.5 cups or less. Men who exercised the most had an 83% lower risk of colon cancer compared to sedentary men. So, guys, get up off the Lazy-Boy, grab a cup of water and your running shoes, and off you go! (*International J of Cancer*, August 1999)

Water and weight loss. Finally, an explanation as to why drinking copious amounts of water while dieting contributes to weight loss. When fluid intake is restricted the resting metabolic rate drops 2-3%. The resting metabolic rate is the rate at which a person at rest burns calories. Since the resting rate accounts for most of the calories burned during the day—even if you get lots of exercise—even a small decline can make it hard to lose weight. Therefore, drinking five to eight glasses of water a day boosts the resting metabolic rate and assists with weight loss.

Water safety around the world. More people die each year from unsafe water than from all forms of violence, including war. More than a billion people—one in every five on earth—do not have access to safe drinking water. The percentage of the population with access to safe water in each of the following countries is: Ethiopia—18%, Sudan—45%, Pakistan—56%, Mexico—72%, USA—99%. (Souce: Water Quality and Health Council: Chlorine Chemistry Council)

WATERCRESS

"Watercress is pleasant enough in a salad or sandwich, but when placed alongside a hamburger it is merely an annoyance." —Fran Leibowitz

WATERMELON

Watermelon. Watermelons were originally domesticated in central and southern Africa somewhere around 6,000 years ago. Watermelon is not only considered a food plant but also a source of water in arid regions. In fact, watermelon has been referred to as a "botanical canteen." Watermelon arrived in the New World with European colonists and African slaves in the early 1600s in Massachusetts. Watermelon seeds were widely dispersed by African slaves in eastern North America. The southeastern states had the best climate and soil conditions to grow watermelon and thus watermelons have been associated, negatively, I might add, with rural African Americans.

Thomas Jefferson grew watermelons at Monticello, Henry David Thoreau grew watermelons in Concord, Massachusetts, and Mark Twain couldn't say enough about the delights of watermelon: "It is chief of this world's luxuries, king by the grace of God over all the fruits of the earth. When one has tasted it, he knows what the angels eat." Indeed, what would a summer be without watermelon-eating contests and watermelon seed-spitting contests?

Wax. Lemons and limes are often waxed to protect them from moisture loss enroute to the store. Before you cut off a piece of the skin for your vodka and tonic, or before you grate the peel to make a tasty zest for a recipe, scrub the peel with a vegetable brush to remove the wax. If you forget to do this don't worry. A little wax will not compromise your digestive system.

Weight gain. And you think you feel fat after a weekend of splurging. The largest dinosaurs could pack on the pounds at a rate faster than you could ever imagine. The apatosaurus, (formerly known as Prince, just kidding), formerly known as brontosaurus, put on more than 30 pounds per *day,* during the adolescent growth spurt. The argentinosaurus, the heaviest dinosaur that has ever roamed the earth, would have gained more than 100 pounds a day during its most rapid growth spurts. And you think your extra 2 pounds over the weekend was tragic. (*Nature,* July 26, 2001)

"Patient's past medical history has been remarkably insignificant with only a 40-pound weight gain in the past 3 days."
Physician notes taken from a patient's hospital chart.

Weight gain and heart disease risk in women. A study in the February 8, 1995 *Journal of the American Medical Association* suggests that women who gain even a modest amount of weight with aging, face an increased risk of heart disease compared to those who manage to keep their weight on an even keel. The findings were surprising.

- Women who gain 11 to 17 pounds over their weight at age 18 run a increased risk of heart disease as compared to peers who had gained fewer than 11 pounds.
- Women who gain 17 to 24 pounds showed a 64% greater risk.
- Women who gain 44 pounds or more face the most serious threat, a 250% greater risk.

Weight gain and hypothyroidism. The issue of weight gain and hypothyroidism has been exaggerated. Although many women would like to blame their weight gain on thyroid problems, hypothyroidism typically isn't the culprit. An underactive thyroid is more often associated with smaller, unexplained weight gains of 5, 10 or 15 pounds. Rarely, if ever, does the weight gain exceed 20 pounds.

Weight gain and television viewing. Researchers as the University of Minnesota School of Public Health followed the habits of more than 1,000 men and women who were trying not to gain weight. They monitored eating habits, exercising habits and television viewing time. By the end of the year, those who spent the most time in front of the TV gained the most weight. Among high-income women, each extra hour of TV viewed per day led to an extra one-half pound of weight gained over the year. Multiply that times 30 years and you have gained 15 pounds just watching TV. YIKES. Well, at least we can blame part of our weight gain on the television. (*American Journal of Public Health*, February 1998)

"Your body is excess baggage you must carry through life. The more excess baggage, the shorter the trip". —Arnold H. Glasgow

---

Weight loss and "fidgeting factor." Investigators at the Mayo Clinic have finally confirmed what many of us have already suspected. Those of us who "fidget" are much less likely to gain weight by overeating.

Nonobese patients in the study were all placed on a 1,000-calorie diet, in addition to their weight-maintenance requirements. Their total energy expenditure was measured through an elaborate technique that took into account things such as basal metabolism rates, postprandial thermogenesis, and volitional exercise. After all of those variables were added, subtracted, multiplied and divided, the remaining energy expenditure was classified as nonexercise-activity thermogenesis, also known as NEAT—the expenditure due to fidgeting, maintenance of posture, and other physical activities of daily life. Two-thirds of the subjects' increases in total energy expenditure proved to be in this category. Moreover, changes in NEAT accounted for 10-fold differences in fat storage and directly predicted resistance to weight gain associated with overfeeding. (Levine JA, Eberhard NL, Jensen MD. "Role of nonexercise activity thermogenesis in resistance to fat gain in humans." *Science* 1999; 283; 212)

"If you want to lose 170 pounds right away, get rid of your husband." —George Burns

---

Weight Watchers. Weight Watchers emphasizes calorie-controlled, high-fiber eating and healthful lifestyle habits. The 1-2-3 success program assigns members a daily food point allotment, which averages 1,250-1,500 calories per day for women. Weekly group meetings with mandatory weigh-in are part of the package. (1-800-651-6000 or www.weight-watchers.com)

"You know you've reached middle-age when your weight-lifting consists merely of standing up." —Bob Hope

---

Wheat bran. In the early 1960s and 1970s, the fiber-rich bran from wheat was fed to cattle. We ate the wheat products without the fiber, the cows ate the fiber-rich bran. What happened? We were constipated and the cows were regular. What's wrong with this picture?

Whole wheat—the whole truth. How do you know that the bread or cereal you buy is whole wheat? (Meaning that it contains the entire layer of the grain including the bran portion). *Read the label.* Ingredients are listed by order of volume, so that first ingredient should be whole wheat or another whole grain. Beware of words like bromated, bleached, and wheat, only "whole wheat" or "100% whole wheat" as the first ingredient is the "real" thing. Most bread made with whole wheat or oats contains two to three grams of fiber per slice.

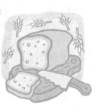

Wishbone. We have all grabbed an end of the slippery little wishbone and made a wish before pulling it apart. But, what does a chicken use a wishbone for? It must have a function in the bird or it wouldn't be there, right? Right. Each end of the wishbone is attached to one of the bird's two scapulae or shoulder bones. Rapid compressions of the wishbone during flight squeezes air back and forth between the two lungs and between various sacs that serve to cool and lighten the bird's body. By squeezing and expanding these air sacs, the wishbone increases the amount of oxygen available to the lungs, a big bonus during the high energy, high oxygen demanding exertions of flight. Seems to be kind of a waste in chickens doesn't it? How many chickens do you see gliding through the air flapping their wings? But all birds contain the wishbone, we're just more familiar with the wishbone from poultry.

Consider the wishbone of the hummingbird for a second. The ten-gram hummingbird uses ten times more oxygen per gram of body weight than the most energetic human. To do this, the hummingbird's heart beats about 1,440 times per minute compared to the heart of the exercising human that beats anywhere from 110-220 beats per minute. This requires a lot of flapping of those hummingbird wings and lots of wishbone compressions!

Wild rice. Actually, wild rice is a misnomer. It is not a type of rice, it is a grass seed native to North America. It is grown in California and Minnesota and shipped around the U.S. to a supermarket near you. It has 70 calories per ½ cup compared to plain ol' white rice that has 110 calories per half cup. It also has some B vitamins. (University of California, *Berkeley Wellness Letter*, Vol. 17, No. 1, October 2000)

Wine. Red wine (purple grape juice) or white wine, what's the difference? The tannins found in red wine are responsible for the inhibition of platelet aggregation and protection from heart disease by reducing the tendency to clot. In addition, red wine contains chemicals known as polyphenols. These chemicals prevent the LDL-cholesterol from oxidizing and forming plaque in the wall of the arteries. How much wine is protective? Two four-ounce glasses per day is all you need for this double-whammy protective effect. In a study of the antioxidant properties of red wine, the antioxidant activity increased significantly within two hours of consumption. Regular consumption could result in a 40% decrease in heart disease in American adults and a savings of $40 billion annually. Sounds like a perfectly healthy excuse for sipping a glass or two in the evening. (Quantum Sufficit, *American Family Physician* 1995; 51(6):1372)

One reason to *never* quit drinking the wine…French researchers have pointed out a possible rebound effect for individuals who stop drinking the alcohol. This rebound effect increases platelet stickiness and therefore increases the risk of clot formation and the possibility of a stroke or myocardial infarction. After depriving rats of alcohol for 18 hours, platelet-clotting responses rose by 124% in those given straight 6% ethanol and 46% in those drinking white wine. However, clotting responses *decreased* by 59% in those given red wine. It appears as if the naturally-occurring compound, tannin, is responsible for preventing this rebound effect.

Do you know what that indentation at the bottom of a wine bottle is called? Answer: a kick or a punt.

"If drinking is beneficial, these findings suggest that those who drink wine in moderate amounts may accrue more benefits than do drinkers of other alcoholic beverages." Gronbaek M et al. *"Type of alcohol consumed and mortality from all causes, coronary heart disease, and cancer."* Annals of Internal Medicine *2000 Sep 19; 133:411-9*

W
249

Wisconsin. The Centers for Disease Control has given the state of Wisconsin the distinction as being numero uno for adult binge drinking. Twenty-three percent of the adults in Wisconsin consume five or more drinks in one sitting.

Witches Brew. Three plants, *Atropa belladonna* (nightshade), *Hyoscyamus Niger* (henbane), and the *Mandragora officinarum* (mandrake), have a rich and vivid history as plants used for poisoning purposes, for soothsaying, for magic and for witchcraft. In ancient Greece, it was believed that inhaling a smoldering henbane plant made one prophetic. (Henbane, by the way, is the plant from which Scopolamine is made, and Scopolamine, as we know it in clinical medicine, induces "twilight" sleep.) In ancient Rome wine was mixed with the deadly nightshade plant to experience hallucinations.

The writings of the Middle Ages are replete with stories of witchcraft and devil worship. None other than Anres Laguna, the physician to Pope Julius III in 1545, wrote one such description of a "green unguent" (ointment) known as Witches Brew: "...a jar half-filled with a certain green unguent...with which they were anointing themselves...was composed of herbs...which are hemlock, nightshade, henbane, and mandrake: of which unguent...I managed to obtain a good canister full...which I used to anoint from head-to-toe the wife of the hangman (as a remedy for her insomnia). On being anointed, she suddenly slept such a profound sleep, with her eyes open like a rabbit (she also fittingly looked like a boiled hare), that I could not imagine how to wake her..."

As the story continued in Dr. Laguna's writings, she was finally aroused 36 hours after her "anointment" with the green stuff. When she was awakened, she appeared to be quite grouchy about being disturbed from her deep sleep. She snapped at Dr. Laguna: "Why do you wake me at such an inopportune time? I was surrounded by all of the pleasures and delights of the world." Upon further questioning, she described the pleasures and delights as vivid episodes of flying and orgasmic adventures. She experienced evenings of debauchery at various banquets, music halls, and dances, where she "coupled with young men" which she "desired the most."

At some point in the Middle Ages it was discovered that if the constituents of Witches Brew were combined with fats or oils they would penetrate the skin and could be easily absorbed through the sweat glands in the axillary areas (armpits) or body orifices (vagina and rectum, being the two that come to mind). You might ask at this point, why the oral route was not considered. Because the potion was too deadly if taken by mouth. Application of the ointment via the armpits or "private parts" allowed the psychoactive drugs to reach the bloodstream and brain without passing through the GI tract and risking poisoning from the metabolic products of liver metabolism.

Numerous writings from the Middle Ages contain statements about the mode of application of the "Witches salves" or "Witches ointments." For example, in the writings of Lady Alice Kyteler in 1324, the inquisitor states: "...in rifling the closet of the ladie, they found a pipe of ointment, wherewith she greased a staffe (i.e., broomstick), upon which she ambled and galloped through thick and thin." Whoopee! In another writing from the fifteenth century records of Jordanes de Bergamo: "... But the vulgar believe, and the witches confess, that on certain days and nights they anoint a staff and ride on it to the appointed place or anoint themselves under the arms and in other hairy places..."

And now, you know the rest of the story. This, my faithful readers, is why so many of the pictures during the period of the Middle Ages, depict the witches riding broomsticks through the sky! Gives new meaning to the witch riding the broomstick at Halloween, doesn't it?

Worcestershire sauce. One of the major claims of Worcestershire sauce is that is it one of the hardest words to say or to spell. Its other major claim to fame is that there would be no Bloody Mary in the world without it. But it was discovered somewhat by accident by two "chemists" who opened a shop in Worcester, England. Their names were John Lea and William Perrins and they named their shop after themselves—Lea & Perrins.

The recipe for Worcestershire sauce was actually a recipe they were asked to make by a customer. The customer had visited Bengal and had returned with the unusual recipe. Lea and Perrins mixed it up and after tasting it they decided it was not fit for human consumption. For whatever reason they did not discard the sauce. They stored the jars of the "mixture" in the cellar and forgot about them. Years later, as they were cleaning out the cellar, they rediscovered the jars of the Bengal recipe. They tasted it again and a star was born! It was delicious the second time around. The liquid had aged and matured. They marketed the concoction, as Lea & Perrins Worcestershire Sauce and it quickly became popular around the world.

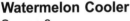

Watermelon Cooler
Serves 8

breakfast · lunch · dinner

- 6 cups waterrnelon pieces, seeded
- 1/4 cup sugar
- 1/2 cup lime juice, fresh
- 4 cups water

In a blender, process the melon, sugar and lime juice.

Strain the mixture through a sieve (pushing all the fruit liquid you can) into a tall pitcher. Discard the pulp.

Add the water, stir and cover with plastic wrap. Chill.

Before serving, mix well and pour into ice-filled glasses.

Nutritional info: 1 serving: Calories 88; Total fat 0.1 gr.; Protein 0.8 gr.; Carbohydrates 21 gr.; Fiber 1 gr.; Sodium 10 mg.

X
is for...
X-Rated

XXX Sugar. No, this isn't about X-Rated Adult sugar! Powdered or confectioner's sugar is granulated sugar that has been crushed into a fine powder with a small amount of cornstarch added to prevent clumping. The XXX's are the designation as to the fineness of the powder and go all the way up to XXXXXXXXXXXX! You'll usually find XXX or XXXX in the baking section of your grocery store.

Xenical (Orlistat). Xenical is a diet drug that interferes with the breakdown, digestion, and absorption of dietary fat in the gut. It is for individuals who have a hard time cutting back on fat intake and who have a Body Mass Index (BMI) greater than 30 or greater than 27 with concomitant medical conditions hypertension, diabetes, or elevated cholesterol.

Xenical inhibits fat absorption by 30%. It does *not* reduce appetite nor does it speed up metabolism. It's not a great weight loss drug, so the search is still on for the optimal drug to help shed those pounds.

"Never eat more than you can lift."
—Miss Piggy

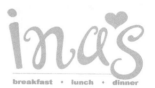

XXX Sugar

Here's a simple icing recipe.
Makes about 1/2 cup

　　1　cup powdered sugar
　1/2　tsp. vanilla
　　milk or orange juice

In a small mixing bowl combine the sugar and vanilla. Stir in 1 tablespoon of milk or juice, adding 1 teaspoon at a time until the icing is smooth and you can drizzle it over a cake.

Nutritional info: Are you kidding?

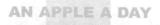

Yam Scam

Yam scam. Let's start with the most important point to make about "The Wild Yam Scam." Yams do *not* contain the hormone progesterone. So, eating a bushel of yams, whether from Mexico or Montana, will not help hot flashes, sleep disturbances, period irregularities, or any other symptoms of menopause or perimenopause. Having said that, let me explain.

Yams contain a compound called diosgenin that can be converted to progesterone, but this conversion can only take place in a laboratory, not in the human body. The body cannot and will not transform the plant hormone into a human hormone. The so-called "natural" progesterone creams are *not* natural. The creams contain an added form of micronized progesterone made in the laboratory by a pharmaceutical company. A compounding pharmacy has the capability of doing this, but this brings us to the second caveat.

Yam cream rubbed on the skin cannot be absorbed in reliable therapeutic doses. Even though natural progesterone is absorbed through the skin, studies have shown time and again, that it is very difficult to achieve therapeutic blood levels with this route of administration.

So, what's a girl to do? You can take "natural" progesterone via the pill route in the form of a drug, Prometrium. Or you can insert a vaginal progesterone gel, Crinone. Both forms are prescription drugs. Steer clear of the over-the-counter creams, lotions and potions. Few of them if any, contain active ingredients. And, for heaven's sake, don't consume massive quantities of wild yams. You'll get a sure-fired case of orange skin but nary a hormone for those hot flashes.

Yogurt. You just can't top a cup of plain fat, low-fat or fat-free yogurt when it comes to calcium (400 mg) and calories (100). That's more than a cup of 1% or fat-free milk. And, like milk, a cup of plain yogurt contains protein, vitamin B12, riboflavin or vitamin B2, potassium, magnesium, and zinc. Unlike milk, yogurt is not fortified with vitamin D. And, individuals who are lactose intolerant can certainly tolerate yogurt because the "live and active" cultures do the work of digesting lactose for you.

All yogurt is made from milk fermented by the bacteria *lactobacillus bulgaricus* and *streptococcus thermophilus.* These "starter" cultures convert lactose, the main carbohydrate in milk, into lactic acid, which curdles milk proteins into the consistency of yogurt.

Most of the health benefits of yogurt are linked to the bacterial cultures. The problem is the survival of these "starter" cultures in the cold cruel world of the gastric environment of the stomach. A pH of 2-3 is not conducive to a long healthy life if you are a *lactobacillus bulgaricus* or a *streptococcus thermophilus.* Some manufacturers have begun to add "probiotics" to yogurt. Probiotics are "live and active" cultures that survive the hostile environment of the stomach pH.

Yogurt as a "probiotic." Probiotics contain live microorganisms that enhance microbial growth in the intestines. Antibiotics destroy the normal flora that inhabit the GI tract. Probiotics inhibit the growth of harmful bacteria, stimulate local immunity, and promote water reabsorption in the colon.

Patients can take them as supplements (Lactinex, etc), or get them from yogurt and other fermented dairy products. Have them choose a brand of yogurt that contains "live and active cultures" such as Dannon, Yoplait, or Colombo. Instruct them to take eight ounces of yogurt twice daily at least two hours after the antibiotic and continue for several days after the antibiotic therapy is finished. Another option is to take Culturelle, 1-2 capsules, each day.

One of the best yogurts available in the U.S. is Stonyfield Farm Yogurt. This brand of yogurt contains six "live and active" microorganisms, which help maintain the healthy bacteria in the gastrointestinal tract and may even stimulate the immune system as an additional bonus. Most other yogurts contain only two "live and active" cultures. (*Environmental Nutrition,* "Best designed functional foods," June 2000)

The "live and active" culture that appears to be most effective in colonizing the GI tract and preventing diarrhea is *Lactobacillus GG,* found in the dietary supplement, Culturelle. It appears to be more effective than *Lactobacillus acidophilus,* found in Dannon, Yoplait, or Colombo yogurts.

Y
256

Just what are the benefits? Improved lactose digestion for starters and, a reduced risk of intestinal infection with the likes of *salmonella, shigella, Listeria, E. Coli* and *Campylobacter jejuni*. In addition, the risk of *H. pylori* is reduced by 18%.

A recent study from the *Journal of Pediatrics* (January 1999; 134;14-20), discussed the benefits of a specific lactobacillus strain GG (also known as L-GG) in the prevention of diarrhea in children between the ages of 6 months and 29 months. A significant reduction in the annual episodes of diarrhea was noted, especially in the nonbreast fed 18- to 29-month-old group.

Various beneficial intestinal microflora are eliminated when antibiotics are taken. Antibiotics that can wreak havoc with the intestinal microflora include the cephalosporins, tetracyclines, Trimethoprim/sulfamethoxasole, fluoroquinolones, macrolides, penicillins, sulfonamides, and isoniazid. Some proponents of probiotics recommend taking them for two to three weeks during and after a course of antibiotics. Give supplements during and after a course of antibiotics if clinical judgment warrants it.

YOHIMBINE

A warning about recommending the "herbal Viagra," yohimbine. Yohimbine, from the bark of a West African tree, has long been described as a "male potency enhancer." The distributors of Yohimbine have also described it as herbal Viagra, however, *buyer beware*. It has not been effective as a sexual enhancer in men with normal sexual function, however, it may have some effect in men with psychological erectile dysfunction. Yohimbine has also been suggested as an antidote to the sexual side effects of the serotonin reuptake inhibitors (SRIs) such as paroxetine (Paxil), fluoxetine (Prozac), citolopram (Celexa), and sertraline (Zoloft).

Studies in rats were quite promising, and in this case it's too bad that human results don't mimic the results of rat studies. Rats fed yohimbine were able to copulate 45 times in 15 minutes. Their female partners were not amused.

Unfortunately yohimbine has a few side effects that can send you straight to the emergency room, bypassing the bedroom. These include increased blood pressure, numerous drug and food interactions (MAO inhibitors and chocolate, aged cheeses, beer, wine, nuts, aged red meats), nervousness, anxiety, tachycardia, hypertensive crisis, and hallucinations.

Yo-Yo dieting. This method of dieting is used by hundreds of thousands of women around the country. Up 10 pounds, down 15 pounds. Up 12 pounds, down 8 pounds—the yo-yo effect. For years experts thought the yo-yo diet was bad for you-you, and that future attempts at losing weight would be much more difficult due to permanent changes in metabolic rates. Fortunately, that's not the case. Metabolism does not change with this type of diet and it's no easier nor is it any harder to lose weight the next time around.

Yogurt Cucumber Salad
Makes 4 servings

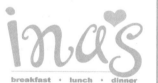
breakfast · lunch · dinner

2-1/2 cups	yogurt, plain, non-fat
3/4 tsp.	garlic, minced
1/2 tsp.	dill, dried
1/2 tsp.	mint, dried
1	cucumber, regular or seedless, grated

Mix together all the ingredients and refrigerate for 1-2 hours before serving.

Nutritional info: One serving: Calories 87; Total fat 0.3 gr.; Protein 8 gr.; Carbohydrates 12 gr.; Fiber 0.5 gr.; Sodium 111 mg.

is for...
Zinc Goodness
it's Over

Zinc (15 mg/day up to 30 mg/day). The best sources of zinc are wheat germ, black-eyed peas, lean beef, seafood, especially crab, oysters and liver.

Zinc and the common cold. Zinc lozenges containing zinc gluconate (Cold-Eeze) have been shown to reduce the length of cold symptoms by half. (*Annals of Internal Medicine* 125: 81, 1996) An important caveat when taking zinc to reduce cold symptoms—taking large doses (greater than 30 mg per day) for a long period of time, can paradoxically weaken the immune system and lower the good HDL cholesterol.

Zinc and immune function. Individuals with zinc deficiency have abnormal T-helper cell function. Since the T-helper cell is responsible for cell-mediated immunity and the immune response to viruses, fungi, cancer cells, parasites and protozoa, replacing zinc to normal levels would boost the immune response to these pathogens and to cancer.

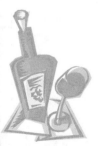

Zinfandel grape. This red wine grape was first used in California to make "jug" wines. However, in the past two decades, fueled by the popularity of zinfandel wines, it has been developed into one of the best of the red varietal grapes and is the most widely grown grape in the state. The zinfandel grape is of European origin but has become known as "California's grape" for two reasons. It has been grown in California since the late nineteenth century and zinfandel wines from that state have been a major contribution to the world of wine. There are both red and white zinfandels, with the "white zinfandel" considered to be a "blush" wine.

Zucchini. The zucchini squash is an American squash that bears the Italian name that is the diminutive of *zucca,* meaning "gourd." Zucchini is also known as summer squash, yellow crookneck squash, and yellow straightneck squash. One-half cup of cooked zucchini slices, with the skin, has 1 gram of dietary fiber, 220 IU of vitamin A (5.5% of the RDA for a woman, 4.5% of the RDA for a man), and 4 mg vitamin C (6.5% of the RDA). One-half cup of yellow squash (either crookneck or straightneck) has 260 IU of vitamin A and 5 mg of vitamin C.

Cold Zucchini Soup
Makes 6 servings

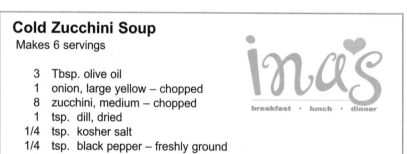

3	Tbsp. olive oil
1	onion, large yellow – chopped
8	zucchini, medium – chopped
1	tsp. dill, dried
1/4	tsp. kosher salt
1/4	tsp. black pepper – freshly ground
3	cups chicken stock, canned, low fat and sodium

In a large saucepan, heat the olive oil over medium heat. Add the onion and sauté, stirring occasionally, until soft – about 5-7 minutes.

Add zucchini, dill and chicken stock and bring to a boil. Reduce the heat to low and simmer uncovered about 10 minutes, until the zucchini is tender. Remove from the heat and cool for 15 minutes.

In a blender or food processor, and working in batches, puree the zucchini mixture. Mix in salt and pepper to taste.

Pour into a large bowl, cover and refrigerate for about 3 hours.

Ladle into 6 chilled soup bowls.

Nutritional Info: 1 Serving: Calories 188; Total fat 10 gr.; Protein 6 gr.; Carbohydrates 10 gr.; Fiber 3 gr.; Sodium 232 mg.

Appendix A

The DASH Diet

Grains and grain products—7 to 8 servings per day
1 slice of bread
½ cup dry cereal
½ cup of cooked rice

Vegetables—4 to 5 servings per day
1 cup of raw leafy vegetable
½ cup of cooked vegetable
¾ cup of vegetable juice

Fruits—4 to 5 servings per day
¾ cup fruit juice
1 medium fruit
¼ cup dried fruit
½ cup of fresh, frozen, or canned fruit

Low-fat or non-fat dairy foods—2 to 3 servings per day
1 cup fat-free or low-fat milk
1 cup low-fat yogurt
1½ oz. part-skim or non-fat cheese

Meats, poultry and fish—2 servings or less per day
3 oz. of broiled or roasted lean meats, skinless poultry, or fish

Nuts, seeds, and beans—4 to 5 servings per week
1/3 cup of nuts
2 Tbsp. sunflower seeds
1½ cup of cooked beans

Added fats, oils, and salad dressings—2 to 3 servings per day
1 tsp. oil or soft margarine
1 tsp. regular mayonnaise
1 Tbsp. low-fat mayonnaise
1 Tbsp. regular salad dressing
2 Tbsp. light salad dressing

Snacks and sweets—5 servings per week
1 medium fruit
1 cup low-fat yogurt
½ cup low-fat frozen yogurt
¾ cup pretzels
1 Tbsp. maple syrup, sugar, jelly, or jam
3 pieces of hard candy

RECOMMENDED FOOD SCORE (RFS)

The following 23 foods are consistent with DASH dietary guidelines. You will receive one point for each of the foods you have consumed at least once in the last week, regardless of the quantity. The maximum RFS is 23. If you score between 14-23 you have a 30% reduction in dying during a 6-year period than if you score between 0-8 points. A high score suggests that you generally watch your saturated fat intake and eat reasonable amounts of fruits, vegetables and whole grains and therefore can significantly reduce your risk of heart disease without making drastic dietary changes.

___ apples or pears

___ oranges

___ cantaloupe

___ orange or grapefruit juice

___ grapefruit

___ other fruit juices

___ dried beans

___ tomatoes

___ broccoli

___ spinach

___ mustard, turnip, or collard greens

___ carrots or mixed vegetables with carrots

___ green salad

___ sweet potatoes, yams

___ other potatoes

___ baked or stewed chicken or turkey

___ dark breads like whole wheat, rye, or pumpernickel

___ cornbread, tortillas, and grits

___ high-fiber cereals, such as bran, granola, or shredded wheat

___ cooked cereal

___ 2% milk and beverages with 2% milk

___ 1% or skim milk

(*Journal of the American Medical Association*, April 2000)

Appendix B

B

USDA Nutrient Database: www.nal.usda.gov/fnic/cgibin/nut_search.pl, *Nutritive Value of Foods,* Home and Gardens Bulletin No. 72 (USDA, 1989)

The International Banana Club and Museum 2524 El Molino Avenue, Altadena, California 91001; 818-798-2272; BananasTB@aol.com or http://www.Banana-Club.com

For more information on how to figure out your BMI check out the website www.nhlbi.nih.gov

C

Hop on to the National Osteoporosis Foundation's web site for more information on calcium and bones: www.nof.org

To contact the American Diabetes Association for a listing of recognized diabetes education programs in your area, call 1-800-DIABETES or visit www.diabetes.org/education/eduprogram.asp

For a copy of the full 670-page report on "Food, Nutrition and the Prevention of Cancer: a global perspective," call the American Institute for Cancer Research at 1-800-843-8114. It's a bargain at $35.00, which also includes shipping and handling. If you prefer, log on to their website for more information at www.aicr.org

Organizations that can offer support and nutritional advice for the gluten-free diet: American Celiac Society (973) 325-8837; Celiac Disease Foundation (818) 990-2354; Celiac Sprue Association/USA, Inc. (402) 558-0600; Gluten Intolerance Group of North America (206) 325-6980

D

Would you like to learn more about the DASH diet? See appendix A for an example of a 2,000 calorie DASH diet, or you can also contact the National Heart, Lung, and Blood Institute, 1-800-575-WELL . Web site:www.nhlbi.nih.gov

E

For more egg-citing information concerning eggs, log on to the American Egg Board's web site at aeb.org

F

Food-borne illness: www.foodsafety.gov, www.fightbac.org; www.cdc.gov.foodsafety; www.cfsan.fda.gov/~mow/intro.html

Check out www.flaxcouncil.ca for all of your flaxseed questions or just for general information on the use of flaxseed as a dietary supplement.

Food Pyramid. If you would like to evaluate your own diet, check out the new USDA interactive website. Go to www.usda.gov/cnpp and click on "The Interactive Healthy Eating Index." See how you stack up to the Food Pyramid and go from there.

G

While you're in Gilroy, California, stop by the Bonfante Gardens Theme Park, the newest of America's theme parks. It features a ride called the Garlic Twirl. For more information on the horticultural theme park, log on to www.bonfantegardens.com.

For information on the glycemic index, hop on line and go to www.glycemicindex.com, www.comm.cornell.edu/gmo/gmo.html — Cornell University's GEO PIE Project, www.cgfi.com — the Center for Global Issues

Checik out tThe USDA laws and regulations governing biotechnology—www.aphis.usda.gov/biotechnology/laws.html

The Council for Biotechnology Information – coalition of corporations that produce GMFs, such as Monsanto, Novartis, and Aventis—www.biowhybiotech.com

The Biotechnology Institute is dedicated to enhancing the understanding of bioscience among lay audiences and in fostering public education collaborations among bioscience companies, universities, and non-profit organizations—www.biotechinstitute.org

H

For information on herbal products for kids, check out www.herbsforkids.com. To find out if an herbal product is legitimate, log on to www.consumerlab.com and look up the products in question.

For more information on heart disease and homocysteine, log on to the American Heart Association's web site: www.amhrt.org

M

For more information on CJD, vCJD, BSE, scrapie and kuru, log on to www.mad-cow.org or www.cdc.gov

O

For more information log on to the web site of the Organic Consumers Association at www.purefood.org. Check it out for lots of links, oodles of information, and resources on topics related to organic food, vegetarianism, and genetically modified foods.

S

The website sponsored by the North American Menopause Society has more information on soy and menopause:www.menopause.org

Websites of Interest

Visit Barb's own web site at: **www.barbbancroft.com**

www.encarta.msn.com Check out Encarta's encyclopedia site and type in "human nutrition." In addition to providing links to more specific nutrition topics, you'll get a refresher course on proteins, fats, carbohydrates, vitamins and minerals, plus explanations of the Recommended Daily Allowances (RDAs) and the Food Guide Pyramid.

Need more info on vitamins and dietary supplements? A great source for information on vitamins and minerals is available through none other that our very own Federal Government's web site **dietary-supplements.info.nih.gov.** It contains over 300,000 references, many with abstracts, from published scientific literature dating from 1996. Dig in.

www.nal.usda.gov This website is the National Agricultural Library (NAL), part of the Agricultural Research Service of the U.S. Department of Agriculture, which is one of the four National Libraries of the U.S. NAL is a major international source for agriculture and related information. This website provides access to NAL's many resources as well as access to its associated institutions.

www.nal.usdalgov/fsrio If you are interested in finding out more about food safety issues and specifics concerning food safety, this is the website for you.

www.foodallergy.org If you want to find out more about food allergies, check out this website. It provides a cookbook with tips for shopping, substitutions and a glossary of ingredient terms. You can also call 1-800-929-4040

www.wheatfoods.org This site is sponsored by the Wheat Foods Council and is a gold mine of information about all sorts of whole grains. You can download facts, recipes, and even have your questions answered by a registered dietician. Just post your question on the message board and it will be answered in a timely fashion.

Appendix C

Interactions with grapefruit and specific drugs
As a general rule, concomitant administration of grapefruit juice with the following drugs should be avoided:

Aprazolam (Xanax), diazepam (Valium) midazolam (Versed), triazolam (Halcion)— antianxiety agents
Carbamezepine (Tegretol)—an anticonvulsant
Cyclosporine (Neoral, Sandimmune)—transplant rejection drug*
The "dipines" or calcium channel blockers with the last name "dipine"—felodipine (Plendil), amlodipine (Norvasc), nisoldipine (Sular), nifedipine (Procardia, Adalat)—antihypertensive agents
Fexofenadine (Allegra)**
Isosorbide mononitrate (Imdur)—antianginal agent
Itraconazole (Sporanox)—an antifungal drug
Lovastatin (Mevacor), simvastatin (Zocor) and atorvastatin (Lipitor)—cholesterol lowering drugs
Nitroglycerine (NTG)—antianginal agent
Quinidine—antiarrhythmic agent
Saquinavir (Invirase), Ritonavir (Norvir)—protease inhibitors for patients with HIV*
Sildenafil (Viagra)—if you don't know what this is prescribed for by now, your head has been in the sand since 1998.
Trazodone (Desyrel) and nefazodone (Serzone)—antidepressants
Verapamil (Calan, Isoptin, Veralan)—antihypertensive agent
Warfarin (Coumadin)—anticoagulant

*In both of these instances, drinking grapefruit juice with the drugs might be beneficial. Increasing the dose of the transplant rejection drug and increasing the dose of the anti-viral drugs in HIV+ patients could provide an extra boost. However, drug levels in each individual would be difficult to monitor, so this is not standard practice today.
**If you are taking the antihistamine Allegra (fexofenadine), and you are not getting the relief from your allergies that you expected, make sure you take it with water and not juice—not *any* juice. Researchers from Canada found that when healthy average Canadians took Allegra with fruit juice, they absorbed only about one-third as much of the drug as when they took it with water. Grapefruit juice had the most powerful effect on absorption, however, other citrus juices also interfered with the ability of the drug to be transported from the intestine into the bloodstream. So, make sure that your patients are educated in the fine art of using water for pill-taking, not juice, coffee, soda, beer, wine or any other liquid.

Appendix D

Glossary

Most medical terms will be defined in the text pages. Here are a few additional definitions that I thought would be of use. All definitions are from Taber's Cyclopedic Medical Dictionary, Philadelphia, PA: F.A.Davis Company, 1997.

Amino acids. Amino acids are the building blocks of proteins and the end products of protein digestion.

Angioplasty. A procedure that reopens narrowed blood vessels and restores forward blood flow.

Anti- is a prefix meaning against, opposing, counteracting

    Anticoagulant—delaying or preventing blood coagulation

    Antiplatelet—destructive to platelets, against platelet function

    Antithrombotic—against clotting, or against the clotting factor thrombin

    Antiarrhythmic—a drug or force that acts to control or prevent cardiac arrhythmias

    Antioxidant—an agent that prevents or inhibits oxidation. Antioxidants are substances that may protect cells form the damaging effects of oxygen radicals, highly reactive chemicals that play a part in atherosclerosis, some forms of cancer, and reperfusion injuries

Apoptosis. Programmed cell death. The cells of the body are programmed to die at certain times.

Arrhythmia. An irregularity or loss of rhythm, especially of the heart

Anaphylaxis (systemic). A life-threatening emergency caused by the response of the immune system to an "allergen" such as shellfish, peanuts, latex, bee stings or penicillin. This reaction of the immune system releases substances from cells in the skin, respiratory system, cardiovascular system, and gastrointestinal system. The clinical signs include itching and hives, respiratory difficulty with shortness of breath, low blood pressure, and nausea, vomiting and diarrhea. If the blood pressure falls low enough, the patient will go into shock. This is referred to as anaphylactic shock.

Carcinogen. Any substance or agent than produces cancer or increased the risk of developing cancer in humans or animal.

Cardiomyopathy. Any disease that affects the heart muscle, diminishing cardiac performance.

Cirrhosis. A chronic liver disease characterized pathologically by liver scarring with loss of normal hepatic architecture and areas of ineffective regeneration.

GABA (gamma amino butyric acid). The brain's principle inhibitory neurotransmitter.

Glial tissue. The nonnervous or supporting tissue of the brain and spinal cord.

Hemochromatosis. A genetic disease marked by excessive accumulation of iron in the body.

Hypertrophy. An increase in the size of an organ or structure, such as the prostate gland (benign prostatic hypertrophy means a noncancerous enlargement of the prostate gland.)

Ketoacidosis. Acidosis due to excess ketone bodies, most commonly seen in type 1 diabetics.

Liquefaction. The conversion of a solid into a liquid.

Myelin is a phospholipid that covers peripheral nerves and central nervous system pathways.

Peristalsis. A progressive wavelike movement that occurs involuntarily in hollow tubes of the body, especially the gastrointestinal tract.

Phytoestrogens. Estrogen-like steroid compounds found in beans, sprouts, fruits, vegetables, cereals, and some nuts. Phyto is the prefix for plant.

Prostaglandins are a large group of unsaturated fatty acids produced in various body tissues. Prostaglandins have a wide variety of functions including vasodilation, influencing vascular permeability, constricting the respiratory bronchioles, causing platelets to clump, boosting gastric acid secretion and inhibiting mucus formation in the stomach, stimulating pain receptors, and inhibiting sleep.

Retinopathy. Any disorder of the retina.

Serotonin. A chemical found in platelets, gastrointestinal mucosa, mast cells, carcinoid tumors, and the central nervous system. Serotonin plays important roles in vasoconstriction, intestinal mobility, nausea and vomiting, obsessive-compulsive behaviors, sleep-wake cycles, depression, and eating.

Thrombolytic. Pertaining to or causing the breaking up of a thrombus, or clot.

Vasodilation. An increase in the diameter of blood vessels, which increased blood flow and lowers blood pressure.

Bibliography

Books

Bratman S. *Health Food Junkies: Overcoming the Obsession with Healthful Eating.* Broadway Books.

Braun S. *Buzz: The Science and Lore of Alcohol and Caffeine.* New York: Penguin Books, 1996.

Carper J. *The Food Pharmacy.* New York: Bantam Books, 1988.

Colburn T, Dumanoski D, Myers JP. *Our Stolen Future.* New York: Penguin Books USA, Inc., 1997.

Dietary Guidelines for Americans, 2000, U.S. Department of Agriculture and U.S. Department of Health and Human Services.

Food Values: Calories. New York, NY. Harper and Row, Publishers, Inc. 1990.

Gardiner, Anne and Wilson, Sue. *The Inquisitive Cook.* New York: Henry Hill & Company, 1998.

Gershon MD. *The Second Brain.* New York: HarperCollins, 1998.

Graedon T, Graedon J. *The People's Pharmacy. city* Mass Market Paperbacks, 1998.

Jones CF. *Mistakes That Worked.* New York: Bantam Doubleday Dell Publishing Group, Inc., 1991.

Kiple KF, Ornelas KC. *The Cambridge World History of Food.* Volume 1 and Volume 2. Cambridge, UK: University Press, 2000.

Lang JH. (Editor). *Larousse Gastronomique.* Crown Publishers, Inc. 1998. New York, NY.

Leibowitz, F. *The Fran Leibowitz Reader,* New York: Vintage Books, 1994.

Lewin RA. *Merde.* New York: Random House, 1999.

Meador C., M.D. *A Little Book of Doctors' Rules.* Philadelphia: Hanley and Belfus, Inc., 1992.

New York Public Library. *The Book of Answers.* New York: Simon and Schuster, 1990.

Nuland SB. *The Mysteries Within.* New York: Simon and Schuster, 2000.

Panati C. *Browser's Book of Beginnings: Origins of Everything Under, and Including the Sun.* Boston, MA: Houghton Mifflin Company, 1984.

Rhodes, R. *Deadly Feasts.* New York: Simon and Schuster, 1997.

Random House Dictionary of the English Language. New York: Random House, 1973.

Rinzler CA. *The New Complete Book of Food.* New York: Checkmark Books, 1999.

Rubin S. *Offbeat Museums.* Santa Monica, CA: Santa Monica Press, 1997.

Schlosser E. *Fast Food Nation.* New York: Houghton Mifflin Company, 2001.

Somer E. *Food and Mood.* New York: Henry Holt and Company, 1995.

Tuleja T. *Curious Customs.* New York: Harmony Books, 1987.

Tyler V. *The Honest Herbal.* Binghamton, NY: Pharmaceutical Products Press, 1993.

Tyler V. *Herbs of Choice.* Binghamton, NY: Pharmaceutical Products Press, 1994.

Watters, P. *Coca-Cola—An Illustrated History.* Garden City, New York: Doubleday & Company, 1978.

Zimmerman BE, Zimmerman DJ. *Killer Germs.* Lincolnwood, IL: NTC/Contemporary Publishing, Inc., 1996.

Zuckerman L. *The Potato: How the humble spud rescued the Western World.* ?city. Faber and Faber, 1998.

Selected Bibliography by Chapter

A

"Alcohol and nosebleeds." (*British Medical Journal* 1994 September 10; 309:640.)

"Alcohol and stroke." (www.prnewswire.com,January 5, 1999; "New York Presbyterian researchers determine that moderate alcohol consumption reduces stroke risk.")

Hobbs WL, Johnson C. "Anorexia nervosa: an overview." *American Family Physician* 1996; 54 (4): 1273-1279.

Leibman B. "Antioxidants: Report sets ceilings." *Nutrition Action Healthletter.* June 2000.

Meagher EA, Oz MC, Pearson TA. "Do antioxidants prevent heart disease?" *Patient Care* 2000 (June 30): 74-93.

Allergies. "Some New Food Allergies Have Nonfood Triggers." *Environmental Nutrition,* May 2000

B

Food and Fitness Advisor. "Diet, Exercise, and Breast Cancer." The Center for Women's Healthcare Weill College of Cornell University. November 1999.

Ross GW, et al. "Association of coffee and caffeine intake with the risk of Parkinson's disease." *Journal of the American Medical Association* 2000 May 24/31; 283:267-9) (World Alzheimer's Congress 2000).

C

Ross GW, et al. "Association of coffee and caffeine intake with the risk of Parkinson's disease." *Journal of the American Medical Association* 2000 May 24/31; 283:267-9.

"The Science of Halloween," Vol. 349, *The Economist, 10/31-1998.*

Grundy SM. "Cholesterol management in high-risk patients without heart disease." *Postgraduate Medicine* 1998; 104(5): 117-129.

Leibman B. "Avoiding the fracture zone." *Nutrition Action Healthletter.* April 1998.

D

"Diabetes: How to cut your risk." *Nutrition Action Healthletter.* May 2001.

Ferzoco LB, Raptopoulos V, Silen W. "Acute Diverticulitis." *New England Journal of Medicine* 1998; 338 (21): 1521-1526.

Dehydration, *Food and Fitness Advisor*, Vol.2, No. 5, May 1999.

Dr. Pepper. New York Public Library. *The Book of Answers.*

Lichtenstein A, Ornish D, Rippe JM, Willett WC. "The best diet for healthy adults." *Patient Care* 1999 (November 15):122-42.

Liebman B. " Diet vs diet: Battle of the bulge doctors." *Nutrition Action Healthletter.* May 2000.

E

Hu FB, et al. "A prospective study of egg consumption and risk of cardiovascular disease in men and women." *Journal of the American Medical Association* 1999 Apr 21:281:1387-94

F

"Low fat, no fat, some fat...high fat? Type of fat, not amount, may be the key." *Environmental Nutrition* April 1998: 21(4).

Kluger J. "What a gas." *Discover,* April 1995: 40-43.

Satish SC. "Belching, bloating, and flatulence." *Postgraduate Medicine* 1997; 101(4):263-278).

Buchanan RL, et al. "The rising tide of food-borne and water-borne infections." *Patient Care* 1997; May 15: 31-72.

Lewin RA. *Merde.* New York: Random House, 1999.

Fuchs CS, et al. "Dietary fiber and the risk of colorectal cancer and adenoma in women." *New England Journal of Medicine* 1999; 340(3):169-175.

G

"Patient Dracula: did a medical condition cause Vlad the Impaler to suck blood and avoid garlic and sunlight? Porphyria symptoms could explain Dracula's behavior." *Medical Post* 7-15-1997.

Jellin JM, Gregory PJ, Butz R, et al. *Natural Medicines Comprehensive Database.* Stockton California: Therapeutic Research Faculty, 2001.
Piscitelli SC, Burstein AH, Welden N, et al. "Garlic supplements decrease saquinavir plasma concentrations." 8th Conference on Retroviruses and Opportunistic Infections, Chicago Illinois, February 2001.
Vuksan V. "Ginseng" *Archives of Internal Medicine* 2000; 160: 1009

H

Jacobs VR et al. "High-density lipoprotein cholesterol as a predictor of cardiovascular mortality in men and women: the follow-up study of the Lipid Research Clinics Prevalence Study." *American Journal of Epidemiology* 1990; 131(1):32-47.
Wood PD et al. "The effects on plasma lipoproteins of a prudent weight-reducing diet, with or without exercise in overweight men and women." *New England Journal of Medicine* 1991; 325(7);461-6.
Suh I, et al. "Alcohol use and mortality from CHD: The role of HDL-C. The Multiple Risk Factor Intervention Trial Research Group." *Annals of Internal Medicine* 1992; 116(11):881-7.
Safeer RS, Cornell MO. "The emerging role of HDL cholesterol." *Postgraduate Medicine* 2000;108(7):87-98.
Stampfer MJ, Malinon MR. "Can lowering homocysteine levels reduce cardiovascular risk?" (editorial) *New England Journal of Medicine* 332; 328, 1995.
"Hamburgers on the grill." *Journal of the National Cancer Institute,* December 2000
Morrison HI, et al. "Serum folate and the risk of fatal coronary artery disease." *Journal of the American Medical Association* 275:1893, 1996.

I

"Cooking with iron." *Environmental Nutrition,* May 2000. Environmental Nutrition Answers Common Questions.
"Concerned about your cookware?" *Environmental Nutrition,* May 2000. Environmental Nutrition Answers Common Questions.

L

"Licorice" *Environmental Nutrition,* March 1999
"AAA Policy Statement on Screening, Treatment and Prevention of Lead Poisoning; Special Medical Report." *Am Fam Phys* 1993; 48(6):1161-1164.
Norman EH, Bordley WC. "Interventions for childhood lead poisoning." *World Ped and Child Care* 1995; 5:107-111.
Leptin. January 1997 Science.

M

Zawada ET. "Malnutrition in the elderly." *Postgraduate Medicine* 1996; 100(1):207-25.
Alzheimer's Prevention Foundation, Dharma Singh Khalsa, M.D., Tucson, AZ.
Hively W. "Worrying about milk." *Discover* 2000 (August): 44-51.

N

Hark L, Deen D. "Taking a nutrition history: a practical approach for family physicians." *American Family Physician* 1999; 59(6): 1521-1528.

O

Shaw GM, Velie EM, Schaffer D. "Risk of neural tube defect affected pregnancies among obese women." *Journal of the American Medical Association* 1996; 275:1093-96.
Werler MM, Lovik C, Shapiro S, et al. "Prepregnant weight in relation to risk of neural tube defects." *Journal of the American Medical Association* 1996; 295:1089-92.

Goodnight SH. "The Fish Oil Puzzle." *Scientific American:SCIENCE & MEDICINE* 1996 (September/October): 42-51.

Weigle DS, Kuijper JL. "Mouse models of human obesity." *Scientific American:SCIENCE & MEDICINE* 1997 (May/June):38-45.

S

Corcoran L, Jacobson M. "Saccharin: Bittersweet." *Nutrition Action Healthletter.* April 1998.

Anderson JW, Quella Sk, Yetley EA. "Sorting out the health claims about soy." *Patient Care* 2000 (December 15);14-30.

Selenium: Anti-Cancer Buzz Brings Star Status. *Environmental Nutrition,* March 1999; 22 (3).

Environmental Nutrition. November 1999; 23(11).

"Environmental Nutrition's Herbal Medicine Cabinet: Top 10 Herbs You Can Trust and 20 You Shouldn't." *Environmental Nutrition.* May 1998: 21(5).

"Soy: modern research investigates an ancient food." The Center for Women's Healthcare Weill Medical College of Cornell University. *Food and Fitness Advisor.* June 2000.

"Is your brain physically fit?" The Center for Women's Healthcare Weill College of Cornell University. *Food and Fitness Advisor.* September 2000.

Freinkel S. "A woman's guide to minerals." *Health* 1998 (October):85-88.

Duffy, Valerie B. "Smell." *Environmental Nutrition.* July 1997.

V

Wolf AM, Wolf A. "Toxicity of vitamins and minerals: how much is too much?" *Hospital Medicine*; 1999 January: 34-38.

Wolf AM, Wolf A. "Evidence-based use of vitamin and mineral supplementation." *Hospital Medicine* 1998 December:53-54.

Hurley J, Corcoran L. "Meals to Go." *Nutrition Action Healthletter.* January/February 1998.

Bikle DD. "A bright future for the sunshine hormone." *Scientific American:SCIENCE & MEDICINE* 1995 March/April: 58-67.

Greenfield MF. "Vitamins and the skin." *Patient Care* 1998 (December 15): 50-71.

Y

Leibman B, Hurley J. "Yogurt: Health food or dessert?" *Nutrition Action Healthletter.* April 1998.

Index

Contributors

Ashley Long

Ashley Long, whose cartoons appear in T*he ABC's of Diet and Disease*, is an 18-year-old artist who lives with her family in Rapids City, Illinois. She graduated from high school with honors in art, English, and journalism, and has been employed as an illustrator, rubber stamp designer, intern, and teaching assistant in a local fine arts program.

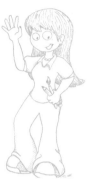

Ashley is attending the College for Creative Studies in Detroit, Michigan to study traditional animation.

Contact Ashley at: JRAK4LONG@aol.com
or email WellWorth Publishing:
info@wellworthpublishing.com

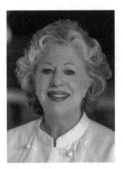

Ina Pinkney

Ina Pinkney, whose recipes grace every chapter, was the chef and owner of the Dessert Kitchen Ltd. for 10 years, supplying private customers, restaurants, caterers, and hotels with desserts. She opened **Ina's Kitchen** in 1991, which quickly became Chicago's premier breakfast restaurant.

During those years, Ina did research and development for recipes for 3 issues of the World Book Encyclopedia's *Christmas Around the World,* the Popcorn Institute, and Quaker Oats. She has taught cooking classes for Marshall Field's, Carson Pirie Scott, the Treasure Island Cooking School, Latin and Parker Schools, and has appeared on local news, cable TV, and radio shows.

Located in the exciting West Randolph Market District in Chicago, Ina's is an urban design with exposed brick walls, beamed ceilings and soft colors. INA'S serves contemporary and updated classic American cuisine for Breakfast, Lunch and Dinner in a casual, quiet and relaxed atmosphere.

Ina has served on the Board of Directors of the Chicago Chapter of Les Dames d'Escoffier and was vice president of the Women's Foodservice Network. She has been featured in articles in the *New York Times*, *Vogue*, the *Chicago Tribune*, the *Chicago Sun-Times*, *Gourmet*, *Midwest Living*, *Restaurants and Institutions Magazine*, and *Nation's Restaurant News*.

Check out Ina's web site at: www.breakfastqueen.com